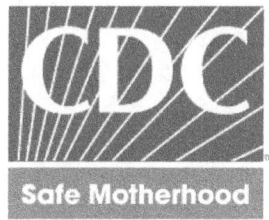

Public Health Surveillance Applied to Reproductive Health

Reproductive Health
Epidemiology Series
Module 1

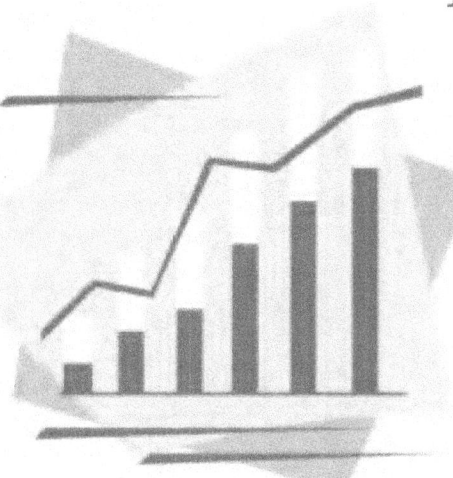

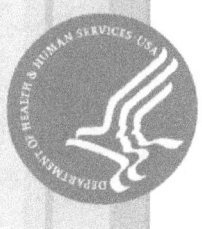

2003

DEPARTMENT OF HEALTH AND HUMAN SERVICES

PUBLIC HEALTH SURVEILLANCE APPLIED TO REPRODUCTIVE HEALTH

REPRODUCTIVE HEALTH
EPIDEMIOLOGY SERIES:
MODULE 1

June 2003

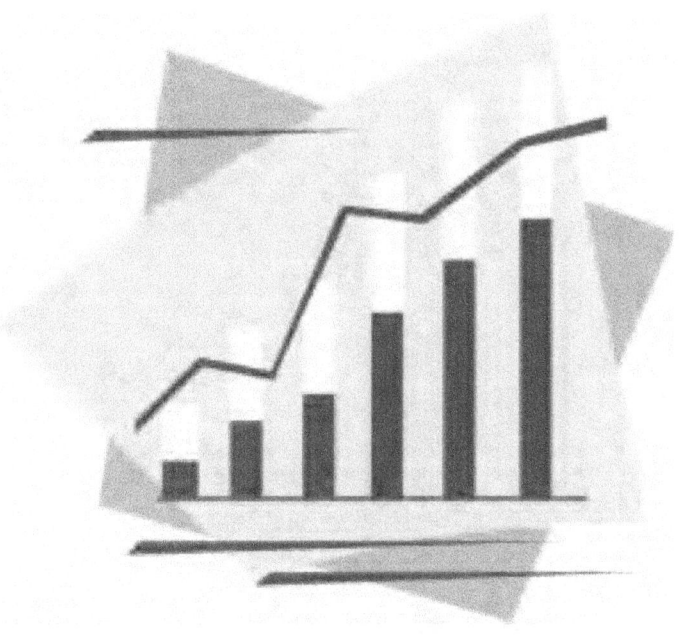

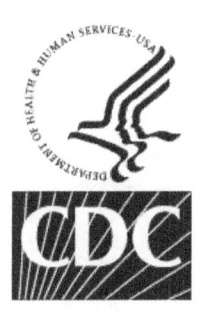

The United States Agency for International Development (USAID) provided funding for this project through a Participating Agency Service Agreement with CDC (936-3038.01).

PUBLIC HEALTH SURVEILLANCE APPLIED TO REPRODUCTIVE HEALTH

Kathryn M. Curtis, PhD
Divya A. Patel, MPH
Tolu Osisanya, MPH

Technical Editors
Isabella Danel, MD, MS
Joy L. Herndon, MS
Florina Serbanescu, MD

U.S. Department of Health and Human Services
Centers for Disease Control and Prevention
National Center for Chronic Disease Prevention and Health Promotion
Division of Reproductive Health
Atlanta, Georgia, U.S.A.
2003

CONTENTS

PUBLIC HEALTH SURVEILLANCE APPLIED TO REPRODUCTIVE HEALTH

LEARNING OBJECTIVES

This module is designed for reproductive health professionals who are interested in conducting and evaluating reproductive health surveillance systems and who need a working knowledge of surveillance in reproductive health.

After studying the material in this module, the student should be able to:

- Define public health surveillance and its components.

- State the goals of public health surveillance.

- List general principles of public health surveillance.

- List the main uses of surveillance data.

- Describe sources of data that can be used for reproductive health surveillance.

- Describe methods and systems useful for conducting reproductive health surveillance.

- Perform basic analysis of surveillance data.

- Discuss the steps in the evaluation of a surveillance system.

- List the various attributes of surveillance systems.

- Describe how surveillance data are linked to public health action.

- Describe how to link health program objectives and indicators to surveillance.

- Use a surveillance grid to plan a reproductive health surveillance system.

- List examples of surveillance systems specific to reproductive health.

Case Study: Increase in Cases of Congenital Syphilis Baltimore, 1993–1996

*B*etween 1993 and 1996, surveillance of congenital syphilis (CS) in the city of Baltimore revealed an increase from 62 to 282 cases per 100,000 live-born infants. Because of this dramatic increase, public health officials assessed the magnitude of the syphilis epidemic in pregnant women in Baltimore and tried to identify ways to increase CS prevention. An assessment of the surveillance system, along with a review of hospital discharge records, yielded the following information:

- All cases of CS found through hospital discharge had also been reported to the CS surveillance system, confirming the completeness of the surveillance system.

- Among 90 women with active syphilis during pregnancy, 62 (69%) delivered infants with CS; 28 (31%) of the infants did not have CS.

- Mothers of infants with CS and mothers of infants without CS had similar demographic characteristics (age, race, marital status).

- Mothers of infants with CS were more likely to have had a third-trimester diagnosis of syphilis, no prenatal care or prenatal care initiated late in the third trimester, and missed opportunities for screening and prenatal care (e.g., spent time in jail or had contact with a social worker or other social service agency).

In response to these findings, public health officials

- Alerted prenatal care and other health providers to initiate syphilis screening and treatment programs for women of reproductive age.

- Initiated a rapid screening and treatment program for detained and arrested women.

- Worked to amend an existing law on syphilis testing during pregnancy to require syphilis testing at 28 weeks gestation or the first visit thereafter to ensure diagnosis in time to prevent prenatal transmission.

Continued surveillance of CS will allow Baltimore health officials to evaluate the effects of these interventions.

Adapted from: CDC. Epidemic of congenital syphilis—Baltimore, 1996–1997. MMWR 1998;47(42):904–7.

INTRODUCTION TO PUBLIC HEALTH SURVEILLANCE

Public health surveillance began centuries ago with the close observation of *individuals* who had been exposed to a communicable disease, in order to detect early symptoms and implement prompt isolation and control measures. This process is now referred to as *medical or personal surveillance (1)*. By comparison, *public health surveillance* is a term used today to describe the process of closely observing health events in *populations*, with a direct and established link to public health action. Over the last 40 years the uses and practices of surveillance have evolved dramatically—surveillance has come to include infection control efforts as well as the monitoring of a wide variety of health events, such as acute and chronic diseases, injuries, environmental and occupational hazards, behavioral risk factors, and reproductive health. Some examples of questions about diseases or other health events that surveillance can be used to answer include the following *(2)*:

- What are currently the most serious health problems?

- What are the emerging health problems?

- Can these problems be prevented?

- How effective and costly are various prevention and control strategies?

- Which prevention and control strategies should be implemented?

- What impact do alternative prevention and control strategies have on health outcomes?

- Do prevention and control strategies need to be modified so program objectives can be met?

- How should scarce economic, material, and human resources be allocated and targeted in order to achieve health goals?

In 1992, the U.S. Centers for Disease Control and Prevention (CDC) convened the International Symposium on Public Health Surveillance, during which surveillance was advocated as an essential part of the global health agenda *(2)*. The symposium focused on the use of surveillance for setting priorities, policy development and program evaluation, effective communication of surveillance information, and the need for capacity building. Surveillance and monitoring of health events are also included among the essential public health functions ranked by the World Health Organization (WHO) *(3)*.

WHO Study of Essential Public Health Functions (rank out of 37)

1. *Immunization*

2. *Monitoring of morbidity and mortality*

3. *Disease outbreak control*

4. *Disease surveillance*

5. *Promotion of community involvement in health*

6. *Monitoring determinants of health*

Source: Bettcher DW, Sapirie S, Goon EH. Essential public health functions: results of the international Delphi study. World Health Stat Q 1994;51:44–54.

Definition of Public Health Surveillance

Public health surveillance is the "ongoing systematic collection, analysis, interpretation of data (e.g., regarding agent/hazard, risk factor, exposure, health event) essential to the planning, implementation, and evaluation of public health practice, closely integrated with the timely dissemination of these data to those responsible for prevention and control" *(4)*. This definition highlights the essential features of surveillance systems, which are the systematic and ongoing collection, analysis, interpretation, and dissemination of data that lead to action and a link with public health practice.

Surveillance systems depend on networks of people and activities to maintain the flow of information and may function at a range of levels, from local to international. Surveillance systems are often considered information loops or cycles involving health care providers, public health agencies, and the public *(1)*. Public health surveillance systems are used to collect descriptive data that identify characteristics of person, place, and time regarding the particular health event under surveillance. In contrast to one-time surveys or epidemiologic studies, surveillance is a process that continues over time. Sometimes, repeated surveys are used to detect trends in the data. Importantly, a surveillance system is not complete without feedback components and a direct link to public health action.

The essential link between public health surveillance data and public health action is the application of these surveillance data to health promotion and disease prevention. Individuals and groups who have the resources to undertake effective prevention and control activities in response to the information provided by the surveillance system need to be included in the dissemination and communication of results from the surveillance system. Health care providers, health agencies, and the public are all responsible for disease prevention and control, and therefore should receive feedback of surveillance information *(2)*. Table 1 illustrates the link between surveillance and public health action for decision making.

Table 1. The Components of Surveillance and Resulting Public Health Action

Public Health Surveillance	Action
Surveillance	**Public Health Action**
Goals & objectives	Priority setting
Collection	Planning, implementing, evaluating:
Analysis	• disease investigation
Interpretation	• disease control
Dissemination	• disease prevention

Adapted from: Principles of epidemiology: an introduction to applied epidemiology and biostatistics. Atlanta (GA): Centers for Disease Control and Prevention; 1992. p. 291.

Principles of Surveillance

An effective surveillance system:

- Addresses health events that are of considerable public health importance; in other words, health events that cause a substantial amount of morbidity and/or mortality and are amenable to practical control or prevention measures.

- Responds to clearly defined objectives.

- Identifies and correctly classifies a large proportion of target health events.

- Correctly reflects the distribution of events over time, place, and person.

- Includes the following components: 1) a clear definition of the health event(s) under surveillance; 2) a clear and logical path for data flow; 3) an adequate knowledge of the population under surveillance; and 4) well-defined and appropriate methods for collection, analysis, interpretation, and feedback of information.

- Results in meaningful and effective public health action based on the data obtained from the system.

- Consists of a simple, flexible, and responsive architecture.

- Promotes a high level of participation of all those involved in the system.

- Provides information in a timely manner so as to enhance relevant public health action.

- Requires justifiable resources to establish and maintain.

An effective surveillance system allows for the integration of epidemiologic, behavioral, laboratory, demographic, and other types of data to provide the information needed by those who must take action *(2)*.

Ethics of Public Health Surveillance

As with all public health activities, practitioners must address the ethical issues associated with surveillance activities. In particular, issues of privacy, confidentiality, and potential need for informed consent are important to resolve when designing a surveillance system. Finally, a surveillance system that only collects data but does not facilitate the use of that data for public health action can be considered an unethical system because it wastes valuable public health resources with no benefit to the public.

In addition to complying with any regulations of the country or institution that is implementing the surveillance system, the following questions can be helpful in addressing ethical issues related to surveillance systems (5):

1. Can you justify the surveillance system in terms of maximizing potential public health benefits and minimizing harm to the public and individuals?

2. Can you justify the use of any identifiers and the maintenance of records with identifiers?

3. Should you elicit informed consent from potential surveillance subjects?

4. Can confidentiality of information collected from individuals be ensured?

5. Have the surveillance protocols been reviewed by colleagues and outside experts?

6. Do you have a plan for sharing data and findings with colleagues, clinicians, the public health community, and the general public?

7. Do you have a plan for ensuring that the surveillance findings lead to action—change practice, target resources and interventions, monitor trends over time, and stimulate other activities to improve the public's health?

PUBLIC HEALTH SURVEILLANCE APPLIED TO REPRODUCTIVE HEALTH

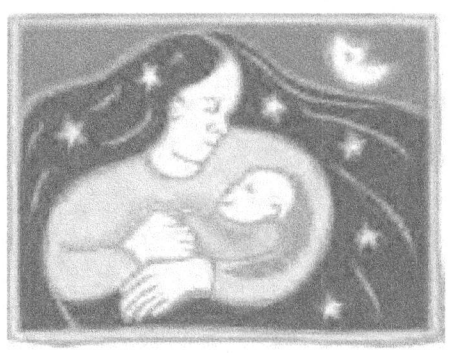

Reproductive health surveillance can be defined as "a component of the health information system that permits the identification, notification, quantification, and determination of events of reproductive health significance for a defined period of time and specified geographic location(s), with the goal of orienting appropriate public health measures for disease prevention and health promotion" *(7)*.

The goal of reproductive health surveillance is to identify or examine ongoing patterns of health events so as to effectively investigate and control the public health events in question, and to prevent morbidity and mortality in a population. Surveillance data are used both to determine the need for public health action and to assess the effectiveness of programs. Reproductive health events that can be tracked through a surveillance system include, but are not limited to:

- Vital statistics (births and fetal deaths).

- Deaths and ill health due to pregnancy (maternal mortality and morbidity) and other pregnancy-related events.

- Infant deaths and ill health.

- Sexually transmitted diseases.

- "Risky" behaviors before or during pregnancy.

- Contraceptive practices.

- Unintended pregnancy.

- Indicators of health services such as prenatal care.

> **WHO Definition of Reproductive Health**
>
> *The World Health Organization (WHO) defines **reproductive health** as a condition in which the reproductive process is accomplished in a state of complete physical, mental, and social well-being, and is not merely the absence of disease or disorders of the reproductive system. It involves the interaction of four main components: 1) the ability, particularly of women, to regulate and control fertility; 2) safe motherhood; 3) infant and child survival, growth, and development; and 4) safety from sexually transmitted disease (6).*

USES OF SURVEILLANCE DATA

Surveillance data are used to monitor health events to determine the need for public health action and to evaluate the effectiveness of programs. It is crucial to understand the uses of surveillance data, their application in decision-making, and their role in identifying research opportunities. Officials responsible for the health of the population are dependent on surveillance data because of the focus on providing information for public health action and a mechanism to evaluate control and prevention programs.

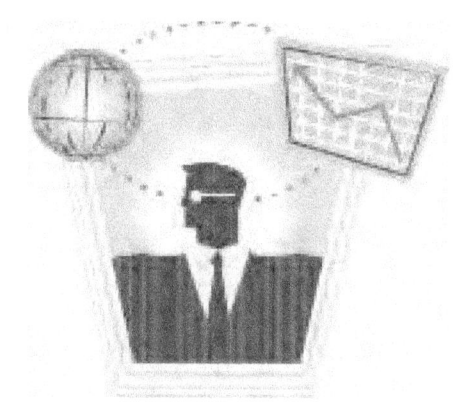

Surveillance data can be used for the following:

Identify the Health Status of a Population

* *Identify new syndromes and infectious agents.* New syndromes have been identified from the reporting, analysis, and interpretation of descriptive surveillance data. For example, researchers noticed unique clinical presentations and characteristics of the sentinel cases of acquired immune deficiency syndrome (AIDS) that suggested a possible connection between these cases. All the AIDS patients who were seen at the University of California at Los Angeles (UCLA) Medical Center in 1981 suffered from the same rare opportunistic infections *(8)*. The UCLA physicians played a crucial role in detecting the presence of a new disease in their community by characterizing the unusual pattern of disease occurrence by person, place, and time.

* *Estimate the magnitude of a health problem.* Surveillance data are used to quantify the magnitude of a health problem or the burden of disease due to a specific cause. These estimates can be used as baseline figures to prioritize public health problems. Table 2 shows estimates of maternal mortality globally and highlights the discrepancies in the magnitude of maternal mortality between more developed and less developed regions of the world.

* *Determine geographic distribution.* By pinpointing geographic areas of higher prevalence of the health outcome of interest, prevention and control resources can be more efficiently

Table 2. Estimates of Maternal Mortality

UN Region	Maternal Mortality Ratio (maternal deaths per 100,000 live births)	Number of Maternal Deaths	Lifetime Risk of Maternal Death, 1 in:*
World	430	585,000	60
More developed regions[†]	27	4,000	1,800
Less developed regions	480	582,000	48
Africa	870	235,000	16
Eastern Africa	1,060	97,000	12
Middle Africa	950	31,000	14
Northern Africa	340	16,000	55
Southern Africa	260	3,600	75
Western Africa	1,020	87,000	12
Asia[†]	390	323,000	65
Eastern Asia	95	24,000	410
South-central Asia	560	227,000	35
South-eastern Asia	440	56,000	55
Western Asia	320	16,000	55
Europe	36	3,200	1,400
Eastern Europe	62	2,500	730
Northern Europe	11	140	4,000
Southern Europe	14	220	4,000
Western Europe	17	350	3,200
Latin America and the Caribbean	190	23,000	130
Caribbean	400	3,200	75
Central America	140	4,700	170
South America	200	15,000	140
Northern America	11	500	3,700
Oceania[†]	680	1,400	26
Australia–New Zealand	10	40	3,600
Melanesia	810	1,400	21

Source: Data from World Health Organization. WHO revised 1990 estimates of maternal mortality: a new approach by WHO and UNICEF. Geneva, Switzerland: World Health Organization; 1996. p. 1–15.
*Lifetime risk of maternal death reflects the chances of a woman's dying from maternal causes over her reproductive life span, usually given as 30–35 years.
[†]Australia, New Zealand, and Japan have been excluded from the regional totals, but are included in the total for more developed regions.

targeted. Geographic patterns may also generate hypotheses about disease etiology and spread (Figure 1).

- *Identify groups at high risk for a health event of interest.* This information is vital for prioritizing health interventions and allocating resources. For example, the Pregnancy Risk Assessment Monitoring System (PRAMS), supported by CDC, compiles data on maternal and child health indicators of health events that occur before, during, and after pregnancy among women who deliver a live-born infant *(9)*. These data can be used by policy makers to assess the status of public health programs in preventing high-risk pregnancies and adverse pregnancy outcomes. Another example comes from CDC's Pregnancy-Related Mortality Ratio (Figure 2). The figure highlights the increased mortality rates among older women and among black women compared with white women.

Monitor Trends in Health Outcomes

- *Identify changes in the occurrence and distribution of disease to guide immediate action for cases of public health importance.* This is especially important at the local level, in the event of an epidemic or an outbreak. For example, the case study in the introduction (p. 2) illustrates the confirmation of an increase in cases of congenital syphilis by the assessment of surveillance.

- *Identify changes in infectious agents and host factors* to assess the potential for future disease occurrence, and to anticipate changes in the natural history of a disease. For example, increases in antibiotic-resistant gonorrhea were detected in the United States in the 1980s. Surveillance enabled public health officials to monitor the spread of this strain. Surveillance data facilitated treatment and prevention activities, indicating the need for modifications to local

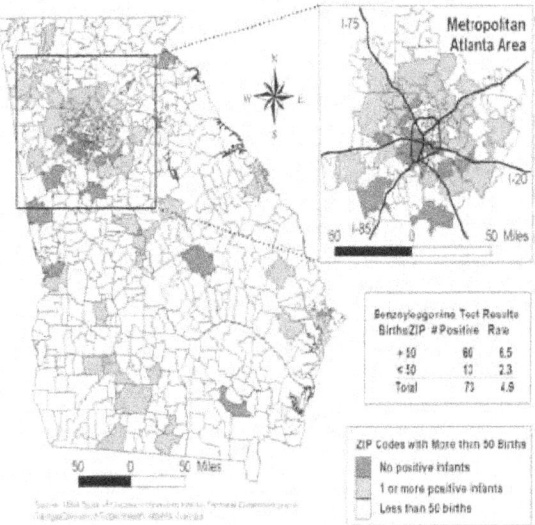

Figure 1. Population-Based Prevalence of Perinatal Exposure to Cocaine—Georgia, 1994

Source: CDC. Population-based prevalence of perinatal exposure to cocaine—Georgia, 1994. MMWR 1996;45(41):887–91. Mary D. Brantley, MPH, MT (ASCP) SI, Centers for Disease Control and Prevention, written communication, March 2001.

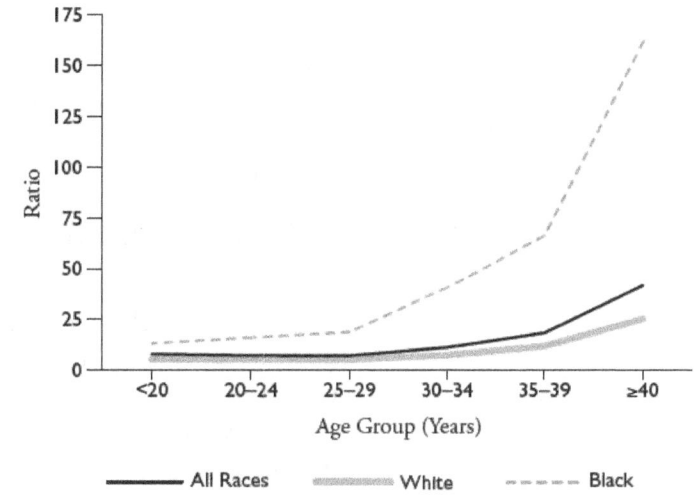

Figure 2. Pregnancy-Related Mortality Ratio,* by Age Group and Race—United States, 1987–1990

*Pregnancy-related deaths per 100,000 live births.
Source: MMWR 1997;46(SS-4):17–36.

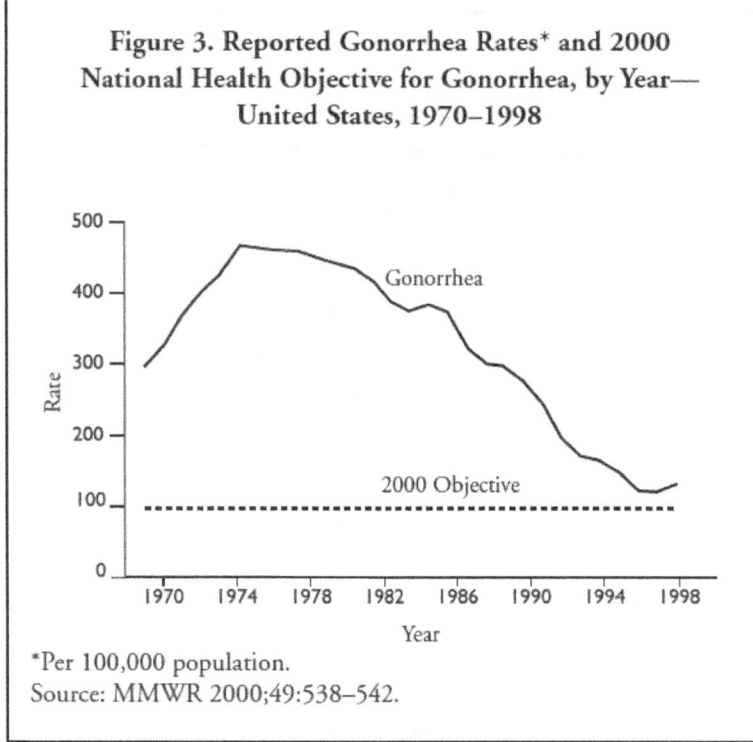

Figure 3. Reported Gonorrhea Rates* and 2000 National Health Objective for Gonorrhea, by Year— United States, 1970–1998

*Per 100,000 population.
Source: MMWR 2000;49:538–542.

guidelines when the proportions of gonococcal strains that met criteria for antimicrobial resistance were greater than or equal to 1% for two consecutive months *(10)*.

- *Determine the etiology and natural history of a disease* by following long-term trends and patterns in populations. The identification of changes in long-term trends is useful information for public health decision makers who need to target strategies and anticipate needs.

Evaluate Public Health Action

- *Guide the planning, implementation, and evaluation of programs to prevent and control disease, injury, or adverse exposure.* National rates of gonorrhea for the United States from 1970 through 1998 (Figure 3) indicate that U.S. gonorrhea rates were dropping and were on target to meet national objectives for the year 2000.

- *Detect the impact of changes in health care practices and public policy.* Data for several maternal health care indicators over time (Table 3) indicate an improvement in maternal health care practices, perhaps due to changes in health care policy in Honduras during this time period.

Set Public Health Priorities

- *Allocate public health resources.* Hemorrhage is the leading cause of maternal deaths in Honduras and the proportion of maternal deaths due to hemorrhage increased between 1990 and 1997 (Figure 4). One strategy for reducing maternal mortality in this setting would be to provide additional resources to reduce the deaths caused by hemorrhage; for example, by upgrading hospital blood transfusion capabilities or by increasing emergency transportation services.

- *Project future needs.* Surveillance data can be used to project future needs, for increasing, decreasing, and stabilizing the need for

Table 3. Maternal Health Indicators: Honduras, 1987–2001

	1987	1992	1996	2001
Any prenatal care in a health facility	65%	73%	83%	85.4%
> 3 PNC visits	—	51%	67%	—
Births in a health facility	41%	46%	54%	54%
Cesarean sections	5.6%	6.4%	6.3%	9.6%

Adapted from: Honduras Ministerio de Salud. Encuesta nacionale de epidemiologia y salud familiar 1996. Honduras: Ministerio de Salud; 1997.

2001 data from: Richard Monteith, Centers for Disease Control and Prevention, written communication, March 2002.

Figure 4. Comparison of Causes of Maternal Death, Honduras, 1990 and 1997

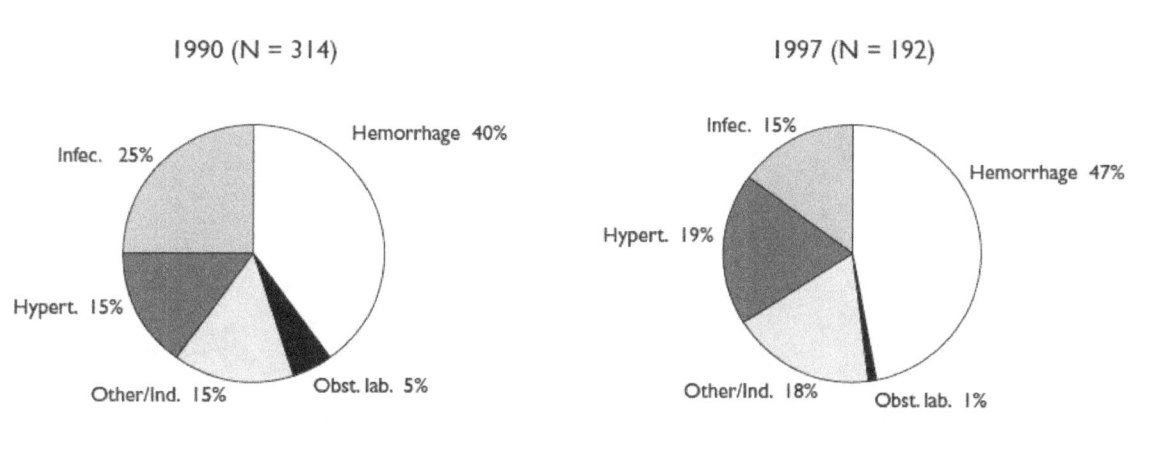

Source: Melendez JH, Ochoa Vasquez JC, Villanueva Y. Investigacion sobre mortalidad materna y de mujeres en edad reproductiva en Honduras. Honduras: Ministerio de Salud; 1999.

---

resources. For example, infant and fetal deaths due to congenital syphilis may be decreasing. Although constant vigilance and resources are needed to screen and treat pregnant women, the resources associated with treating infants with congenital syphilis will decrease. At the same time, perhaps, infant deaths due to other causes may still be high, and resources can now be diverted to new interventions to prevent other causes of infant mortality.

Provide the Basis for Epidemiological Research

- *Generate hypotheses and stimulate research.* Because surveillance data describe a current health situation or changes in the health situation over time, these data can be used to generate hypotheses about the causes and predictors of disease. For example, one can hypothesize that the high proportion of maternal deaths in Honduras due to hemorrhage might be related to health care services for blood transfusions: women may have difficulty accessing these services because of lack of emergency transportation, blood may not be readily available, the time it takes to begin the transfusion may be too long, and the health care system may have other problems. From these hypotheses, an analytic study can be designed to identify the specific causes and predictors of maternal deaths due to hemorrhage, and appropriate interventions can be implemented.

SOURCES OF DATA FOR PUBLIC HEALTH SURVEILLANCE

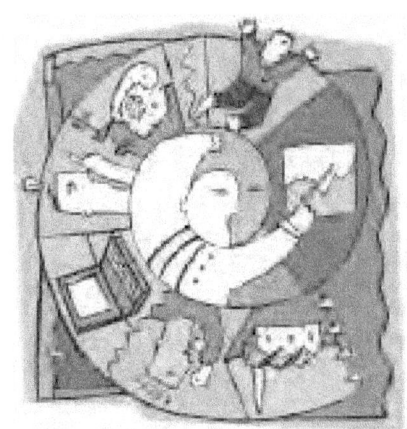

In many instances, analysis of routinely collected data will provide the basis for assessing the public health impact of a particular health event. Routinely collected data provide several sources from which information can be obtained for public health surveillance applied to reproductive health issues. The selection and appropriate use of data from these sources depend primarily on the nature and scope of activities to be monitored.

Vital Statistics

The vital statistics of birth, death, marriage, and divorce are collected routinely in some countries and are a cornerstone of surveillance in both developed and developing countries *(11)*. However, medically certified information on deaths is available only for less than 30% of the 50.5 million deaths that occur every year *(12)*. Vital statistics are particularly important since, in many countries, they are the only form of health-related data available in a standard format and, thus, can be useful for global comparisons. Uses of vital statistics include the following:

- Monitoring long-term trends.

- Identifying differences in health status within racial or other population subgroups.

- Assessing differences by geographic area or by occupation.

- Monitoring illnesses and deaths that are considered preventable.

- Conducting health-planning activities.

- Generating hypotheses regarding etiology or correlates of disease.

- Monitoring progress toward achieving improvements in the health of the population.

Although the usefulness of vital statistics in surveillance varies by health event, in general, vital statistics are more useful for conditions that are easily recognized at the time of birth or death. Mortality rates derived from vital records will most closely approximate the true incidence for easily diagnosed conditions with a short clinical course, and for conditions that are usually fatal.

In the United States, certain states include additional information on perinatal risk factors on their birth certificates as a way to improve surveillance for perinatal events. Birth certificate information can be used, for example, to determine the extent to which women in the

United States received delayed prenatal care or no prenatal care. Some states link information from infant death certificates with maternal characteristics such as age, health status, and race for the surveillance of adverse reproductive health outcomes. Collection of this additional information in turn supports health planning and targeting of services *(11)*.

The quality of vital statistics data depends on several factors, including the completeness of vital registration, the accuracy of data provided on certificates, and the translation of information into computerized data. Registered events tend to differ from those that are not registered. For example, deaths of women in urban areas or who have received better medical care are more likely to be registered than are deaths among women in rural areas or among those who have not received medical care *(7)*. Furthermore, delays in the production of final vital statistics at a national level are common, even though birth and death certificates are filed shortly after the event occurs. Death certificates cannot provide accurate information on the impact of diseases with low case-fatality rates or long latency periods. Despite these limitations, vital records serve an important function in providing information for surveillance of a wide range of health events at local, national, and international levels. Routine analysis of data obtained at birth and death may point to areas in need of further investigation.

Morbidity Data

Morbidity data, or data on diseases and other health events, are obtained from several sources, including notifiable disease reports, hospital data, outpatient and special clinics data, and laboratory data. Registries are another valuable source of health data.

Notifiable disease reports. Health care providers are required to report certain health events occurring within a geopolitical boundary (county, state, province, etc.). Requirements to report health events vary from place to place, depending on health priorities and policies. In general, a disease is designated as notifiable when the link between case report and public health action is clear (i.e., the report of a case of the health event under surveillance leads the health authorities to take certain measures) *(13)*. Sexually transmitted diseases such as chancroid, gonorrhea, syphilis, HIV infection, and AIDS are required to be reported by law in many places. In some areas, abortions and maternal deaths are included in the list of reportable events.

In general, persons obligated to report known or suspected notifiable conditions include physicians, dentists, nurses, and other health professionals, medical examiners, and administrators of hospitals, clinics, nursing homes, schools, and nurseries. In some cases, laboratories and the general public are required to report notifiable diseases. These reports are routinely used by health agencies at all levels for public health surveillance—local, national, and global.

Hospital data. Many hospitals maintain discharge records for administrative and financial purposes. Local and national surveillance systems can make use of these data by collecting information from samples of hospitals for surveillance of a wide range of pregnancy-related events, including birth defects, infant deaths, unintended pregnancy, and maternal morbidity and deaths. Pertinent information available through hospital records may include demographic information, diagnoses, length of hospital stay, outcome, and other patient information that can be reported without identifying individuals. Along with information on burden of disease, this information may also provide important data on health activities.

A disadvantage of using hospital data is that they are facility-based and, thus, population-based rates usually cannot be estimated. Hospital data are most useful for conditions or procedures for which patients are typically hospitalized, for example, cesarean sections, but less so for conditions for which many patients are treated outside a hospital setting, for example, pelvic inflammatory disease. Another disadvantage is that fee-for-service hospitals or ones that serve patients with a certain type of insurance may admit mainly economically advantaged people. Such hospitals may have lower rates of severe illnesses or deaths than the rest of the community. Hence, rates derived from hospital data must be interpreted with caution before they can be generalized to the overall population.

Outpatient and special clinics data. Information from special outpatient clinics can be especially useful in reproductive health surveillance of sexually transmitted diseases (STDs) and pregnancy-related outcomes. Outpatient data also are facility-based and thus usually cannot be generalized to the population.

Laboratory data. Laboratories can be a useful source of surveillance data in reproductive health epidemiology, especially for diseases in which laboratory confirmation is essential for diagnosis (e.g., confirmation of HIV infection). Laboratory-based surveillance is an important component of the prevention and control of reproductive tract infections (RTIs). The traditional approach to diagnosis and treatment of RTIs is through laboratory diagnosis to determine the etiologic agent causing infection. In developed countries, laboratory

Reproductive Health Epidemiology Series

tests are used to confirm symptomatic infections, as well as detect asymptomatic infections, and thus provide data for epidemiological surveillance and monitoring of disease sensitivity to antibiotic treatment (antibiotic resistance).

Registries

A registry serves as a listing of all occurrences of a disease or category of disease (such as cancer, birth defects, or immunization) within a defined area *(4)*. Information is collected from multiple sources (e.g., hospital-discharge data, treatment records, pathology reports, and death certificates) and is linked for each individual over time (e.g., the immunization schedule for a particular child over time and across multiple health care providers). This linkage of individuals over time is unique to registries. Registries have been used to monitor a wide range of health events and have identified opportunities for public health prevention and control activities.

Registries can be facility- or population-based, although population-based registries from which incidence rates can be calculated are generally more useful. However, even if population at risk is not known, facility-based registries can be useful for a variety of activities including descriptive analyses and assessment of treatment effectiveness. The main limitation of registries is that high-quality data collection systems are expensive to set up and maintain and, thus, are generally not available in all geographic areas *(11)*. Also, the complexity of the data collection process makes rapid turnaround of data difficult.

Surveys of Reproductive-Age Women and Household Surveys

Information that can be obtained from surveys includes disease status, behaviors associated with disease, risk factors, and health services data. Reproductive health surveys can be either one-time, cross-sectional surveys, or large-scale, periodic surveys. Population-based information for non-notifiable diseases is often obtained solely through the use of surveys of individuals, which can capture cases that are not seen at a health facility. One-time surveys do not provide information that can be used for assessing trends; ongoing or periodic surveys are more useful for surveillance purposes because rates can be monitored over time in a specific region.

Reproductive health surveys provide high-quality data and are routinely conducted by developed countries; however, the expense of conducting such surveys is a serious limitation for developing countries.

Community Identification

Community identification of health events occurs when persons sometimes referred to as "key informants" report information from the community to the health sector (7). Key informants may be traditional birth attendants, village health workers, village leaders, or simply well-connected individuals in the community. For example, maternal deaths that occur in a community may not be reported to a health facility and therefore would not be counted in a facility-based surveillance system. Maternal deaths occurring outside the health system must be identified and investigated because these women often die from different causes than do women who die in hospitals. The community identification approach is important for situations in which a significant proportion of health events do not occur within the health care delivery system and, thus, are not identified through any of the other surveillance methods discussed earlier.

In some settings, estimates of reproductive health events cannot be obtained through direct methods of measurement. The *sisterhood method* is an indirect method of community identification of maternal deaths that makes use of information on maternal deaths obtained by the addition of questions to demographic or community-based household surveys (14). This method, in which a representative sample of adults is asked questions regarding the survivorship of their sisters, provides basic information for the calculation of women's lifetime chances of death from maternal causes. The sisterhood method requires smaller sample sizes than traditional methods and is relatively easy to use in the field.

One of the main problems with the sisterhood method is that it yields no information on the causes or circumstances surrounding the maternal deaths. Furthermore, the method is highly dependent on the prevalence of maternal mortality in the population. This method relies on the idea that siblings maintain contact throughout their lives. This assumption may not be true in settings where women leave the maternal home upon marriage and perhaps migrate to other parts of the country. The sisterhood method tends to underreport early pregnancy deaths, especially those related to abortion or those that occur among unmarried women. Moreover, the sisterhood method can only give a retrospective estimate for the Maternal Mortality Ratio for the past 10 years (15). Nevertheless, the sisterhood method is useful for deriving population-based estimates of maternal mortality in areas where the alternative data sources and approaches to estimation are inadequate, such as areas with poorly maintained or nonexistent vital registration systems.

TYPES OF SURVEILLANCE SYSTEMS

Comprehensive Versus Sentinel Reporting

Comprehensive reporting systems collect information on all cases of a particular health event under surveillance. Routinely collected data on patient care are aggregated on a regular basis and reported. Routine patient care data collection usually includes the whole spectrum of health events seen by the health facility and may include hospital records, home visits, and outreach efforts by health workers. Other sources of comprehensive data for a surveillance system are notifiable disease reports and reproductive health surveys. Since comprehensive reporting provides a wide range of information to the collecting agency, careful scrutiny may be required to identify important trends and changes. Comprehensive reporting systems are commonly used in developing countries, where resources for data collection targeted toward particular health events may be extremely limited.

In contrast, *sentinel surveillance* monitors key health events through selected sites, geographic areas, events, providers, or vectors *(16)*. In this system, selected health facilities are designated as *sentinel sites* and are required to report the health event under surveillance. Although sentinel sites may be obtained from a sample, usually they are chosen because of the likelihood of observing the particular health event at that site and for their cooperation in reporting. Sentinel surveillance encompasses a wide range of health activities for the purpose of obtaining timely information.

In a sentinel system, data typically are reported weekly so that outbreaks and other unusual health events can be detected quickly. Since fewer sites are involved, data collected from sentinel sites are usually more accurate and complete, and data collection is less expensive than in comprehensive surveillance systems. The information obtained from sentinel systems, however, is usually not representative of the general population and is often insufficient to calculate rates and ratios.

Population-Based Versus Facility-Based Systems

Population-based is a term used to describe information collected for all persons in a certain geographic unit, as opposed to *facility-based* information, which may represent only persons from the catchment area of a given health facility. Population-based surveillance is especially important in many developing countries because of disparities in access to health facilities and health status between urban and rural areas. Methods of population-based surveillance include vital registration, periodic reproductive health surveys, and surveillance at the local level (i.e., the lowest level of the health system). *Facility-based* surveillance may include exit interviews, focus groups, and reviews of health clinic records, and supervisory and evaluation reports. Focus groups are often used as a first step in generating ideas about why events and behaviors occur and are useful in the design of surveillance systems *(1)*. *Exit interviews* entail interviewing patients who have finished their visits at health facilities. Exit interviews are ideal for measuring progress at the local level and can be used to collect information on process indicators of health objectives, health risks, health behavior, and health interventions *(17)*.

An important consideration in the design of surveillance systems is that facility-based systems generally do not include cases outside the health care delivery system. For example, a considerable percentage of women in Tanzania go through labor and delivery at home; therefore, a facility-based surveillance system of emergency obstetric complications will represent only a certain segment of the population and may not yield accurate information about labor and delivery complications that can be extrapolated to the population.

Primary Versus Secondary Data

Data that are collected for the purposes of surveillance are called *primary data*, and data that are collected for other reasons (i.e., administrative and financial records) but used for surveillance purposes are called *secondary data*. Although most surveillance systems collect data expressly for the purpose of supporting that specific surveillance effort, secondary data sets are increasingly being used in surveillance *(2)*. Secondary data sets, which may include data from community records and administrative data, usually differ from primary data sources in a number of ways. Secondary data can be an efficient and cost-effective source of surveillance data. Secondary data generally are not available on a timely basis, however, and thus are usually more useful for long-term rather than short-term interventions. Furthermore, all the desired health and sociodemographic information may not be included since the data were not primarily collected for the purposes of surveillance. For example, health maintenance organization data systems have primarily been used for cost accounting. Recently, these large data systems have been used to investigate the adverse reactions to vaccines and to study the cost-effectiveness of family planning services in preventing the high costs of unintended pregnancy.

Passive Versus Active Surveillance

Primary surveillance data collection systems are usually classified as passive or active *(18)*. *Passive*, or *provider-initiated*, surveillance is a form of data collection in which health care providers send reports to a health department based on a known set of rules and regulations. Most routine surveillance relies on passive reporting, in which health care providers report notifiable diseases on an individual case basis to the local level. Surveillance of infant deaths in the United States offers another example of a passive reporting system, in which death certificates are forwarded to the U.S. Centers for Disease Control and Prevention with designated International Classification of Diseases (ICD) codes. Passive systems are often limited by their lack of complete and representative data. They may not be sensitive enough to detect outbreaks. The advantage of passive systems is that they require less personnel to maintain than do active systems, and thus are less expensive.

Given the shortcomings of passive surveillance systems, more active systems may be necessary for conditions of particular public health importance. *Active*, or *health department-initiated*, surveillance involves regular outreach and routine solicitation of reports from potential reporters to enhance the reporting of specific diseases or conditions. In settings of limited resources, active surveillance is often used for short periods for very discrete purposes, such as the elimination of a particular condition from a population. Active surveillance can be used to assess the representativeness of passive reports, enhance the completeness of reporting of specific conditions, or supplement epidemiologic investigations.

COMPONENTS OF THE SURVEILLANCE PROCESS

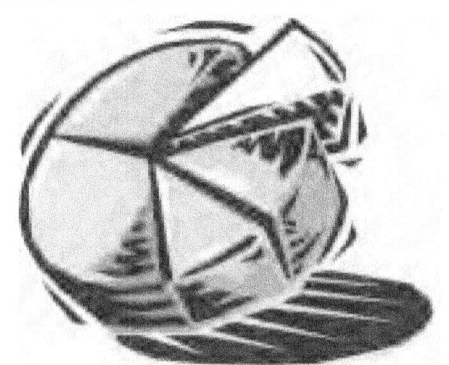

The process of surveillance consists of five main components: setting goals and objectives, data collection, data analysis, interpretation of data, and communication and dissemination of surveillance information that is directly linked to public health action.

Setting Goals and Objectives: Surveillance Based on Health Objectives and Program Indicators

Identifying measurable health objectives, assigning them priority, and linking the design of the surveillance system to those objectives will produce a closer connection between the process of surveillance and public health action *(17)*. It is useful to start with the end in mind and decide on what public health action you want to take; what decisions do you need to make about a particular health problem? The resulting surveillance system is more relevant to the users of the information, which enhances the usability and effectiveness of the system. Because of the inherent relationship between surveillance and health programs, the surveillance process helps in designing and refining health intervention programs, resulting in an efficient use of resources.

Indicators are useful in measuring progress toward predefined health objectives, as well as evaluating the health objective itself. An indicator is a measurement that, when compared with either a standard or desired level of achievement, provides information regarding a health outcome or management process. Indicators can serve as markers of progress toward improved reproductive health status. (See "Useful Indicators in Reproductive Health Epidemiology" to the right.) An indicator can either be a direct measure of impact, or an indirect one, which measures progress toward specified program goals. Indicator data are collected periodically over time to track progress toward system objectives. *Impact* indicators provide information on the end result, but do not provide insight into how the outcome was achieved. For this reason, combining impact indicators with *process* (program activities) and *outcome* (results of those activities) indicators provides the best information to evaluate a surveillance system.

The issue of classification of indicators is widely debated, and definitions vary among different organizations, but process, outcome, and impact indicators are the main focus of this discussion. Process indicators are generally easier to measure than outcome or impact indicators.

Useful Indicators in Reproductive Health Epidemiology

Impact Indicators: Reflect changes in the primary health event of interest (i.e., morbidity, mortality) and other health outcomes.

Outcome Indicators: Reflect changes in knowledge, attitudes, behaviors, or the availability of necessary services that result from program activities.

Process Indicators: Specify the actions needed for program implementation in order to achieve the intended outcomes.

Adapted from: Reproductive health in refugee situations: an inter-agency field manual. Geneva, Switzerland: United Nations High Commissioner for Refugees; 1999.

However, process indicators are limited in that they do not measure the effectiveness of the process, nor do they measure the event of primary interest *(15)*. Thus, process indicators may not necessarily correlate with outcome measures. Accordingly, although process indicators are useful in the short term, outcome and impact measures ultimately must be used to measure actual changes in health status.

For each predefined health objective, the indicator for evaluating that objective should also be defined, as in the following example:

Table 4. Example of Types of Objectives and Indicators in Reproductive Health

	Program Objective	Indicator	Definition
Process indicator	100% of pregnant women will be screened for syphilis before delivery	Coverage of syphilis screening	$\dfrac{\text{Number of women delivering in the specified time period who had been tested for syphilis during the pregnancy}}{\text{Number of live births in the specified time period}} \times 100$
Outcome indicator	Reduce the percentage of pregnant women who test positive for syphilis at delivery from x% to (x – n)%	Syphilis infection among pregnant women	$\dfrac{\text{Number of pregnant women screened for syphilis in the specified time period who tested positive for syphilis}}{\text{Number of pregnant women who were tested for syphilis at delivery in the specified time period}} \times 100$
Impact indicator	Reduce the perinatal mortality rate from y% to (y – n)%	Perinatal mortality rate	$\dfrac{\text{Number of deaths in the perinatal period (22 weeks gestation through 7 days of life) during a specified time period}}{\text{Total number of births (live births plus fetal deaths) during the same time period}} \times 1{,}000$

Adapted from: Reproductive health in refugee situations: an inter-agency field manual. Geneva, Switzerland: United Nations High Commission for Refugees; 1999.

The purpose of linking surveillance to health objectives is to reinforce the concept that surveillance is a system that uses information from multiple sources to impact health status, rather than simply the reporting of disease. Furthermore, linking assists planners to think creatively in efforts to build a surveillance system to measure all priority health objectives.

Data Collection

The sources of data for public health surveillance and methods of data collection have been described in previous sections. In general, there are certain points to bear in mind regarding data collection. First, sources of data and methods of collection should be pretested to ensure feasibility. The training of personnel involved in data collection is an important step in establishing a surveillance system. Data collection instruments should ascertain the minimum information required for surveillance of the health event in order to enhance the quality of data and avoid an additional burden on the health system. Each element of data collected by surveillance should have a clearly demonstrated use *(2)*.

Routine methods of collecting data in a system can be cross-checked periodically with other methods to enhance completeness of data; for example, notifiable disease reports can be supplemented with information from surveys or sentinel reporting. The instruments used for data collection should have a standardized format to facilitate data analysis and comparison of results from other surveillance systems or surveys. Standardizing the format of data collection systems allows for ease of data entry with minimal errors. Use of a standardized format is becoming more important with the shift to applications of information technology to public health issues. Depending on the resources of the particular region, this shift may be either currently relevant or may occur in the future as resources become available.

Analysis of Surveillance Data

The ability to effectively analyze, interpret, and present surveillance data is an important skill for the public health worker. Regular and systematic collection of surveillance information allows the description of health events over time in the population under surveillance. In conducting an analysis, surveillance data are usually compared with an expected value, as well as with baseline information. Thorough analysis includes determination of both actual numbers and rates. As with other descriptive epidemiologic data, surveillance data are usually analyzed in terms of time, place, and person *(1)*.

Time. Description by time is an important means of detecting trends in the health event under surveillance. The comparison of the number of case reports received during a particular interval (i.e., days, weeks, months) may help to identify sharp changes in case counts within the time interval. Comparing the number of cases for a current time period with the number reported during

Public Health Informatics

*Public health informatics is the **application of information science and technology to public health practice and research** (19). This definition of public health informatics encompasses more than computerizing public health information. It is the capability of **available** technologies to manage information—whether those technologies include pencil and paper, handheld calculators, computers, multimedia applications, or a network of global telecommunications (20). The goal of public health informatics is to "speed and simplify the conversion of hypotheses about the distribution and determinants of diseases in populations into usable information, and help to disseminate new knowledge in ways that will support public health practice" (19).*

Public health informatics can be applied to several components of surveillance (20).

Recording and reporting of cases. *The completeness of case reporting depends largely on the amount of effort it takes for the health practitioner to record and report the health event of interest, and the subsequent steps needed to continue the reporting process at all levels of the surveillance system. Two key concepts in enhancing reporting are **standardization** and **integration**. By using standardized classification systems for reporting health-related data (e.g., International Classification of Diseases, tenth revision [ICD-10]), surveillance data can be efficiently reported at all levels of the surveillance system. Standardized, structured record formats and variable definitions for reporting health-related data allow for flexibility in local data collection systems (e.g., different software applications, additional variables of interest at the local level), while creating an aggregate, integrated national database of health events.*

Data transmission. *The technologies associated with public health informatics facilitate the transmission of raw surveillance data through electronic transfers, telecommunications, and computer connectivity. The use of the Internet is increasing at all levels of surveillance, beginning with individuals entering their own personal information into Internet-based data systems.*

Analysis of data. *The use of a computer for analysis of surveillance data is critical for any but the most simple systems, and new technologies are changing the way analysis is done. A primary example is the use of geographic information systems (GIS) to map and analyze changes in the spatial distribution of health events.*

Reporting and disseminating surveillance findings. *New informatics technologies have greatly increased the accessibility of surveillance findings through electronic transfer of reports, Internet access, and multimedia presentations. Additionally, new methods of presenting data in charts, graphs, and maps can enhance the visual perception of burden of disease and changes in disease trends over time. These visual displays can be highly effective in presenting surveillance data to decision makers, who can then rapidly take public health action.*

The key to developing an effective surveillance system is making the best use of the available technologies and looking to the future to integrate new technologies where they will be most helpful. In designing and implementing any surveillance system, public health workers must address the following questions (20):

1. Which specific component tasks of public health surveillance can informatics technology help to perform more quickly, easily, and accurately?

2. For each task, which informatic functions are appropriate, useful, and applicable?

3. Which capabilities of this technology have already been put into use or are under development?

4. What potential uses of informatic technology can we identify now?

In countries with limited resources, a well-planned and -managed paper record system may continue to be the most efficient reporting system available. However, "as surveillance information systems are implemented, every effort should be made to incorporate standardized processes for system connectivity and integration, protocols for data exchange and information access, core health data elements, and standard classification schemes" (21).

Further reading and information

Friede A, Blum HL, McDonald M. Public health informatics: how information-age technology can strengthen public health. Annu Rev Public Health 1995;16:239–52.

Groseclose SL, Sullivan KM, Gibbs NP, Knowles CM. Management of the surveillance information system and quality control of data. In: Teutsch SM, Churchill RE, editors. Principles and practice of public health surveillance. 2nd ed. New York: Oxford University Press; 2000. p. 95–111.

Kilbourne EM. Informatics in public health surveillance: current issues and future perspectives. MMWR 1992;41:S91–S99.

Yasnoff WA, O'Carroll PW, Koo D, Linkins RW, Kilbourne EM. Public health informatics: improving and transforming public health in the information age. J Public Health Management Practice 2000;6:67–75.

Division of Public Health Surveillance and Informatics, CDC: http://www.cdc.gov/epo/ dphsi/index.htm

Health Informatics Worldwide: http://www.imbi.uni-freiburg.de/medinf/mi_list.htm

International Medical Informatics Association: http://www.imia.org/

the same interval in previous years may help determine seasonal patterns of the health event. Graphing the occurrence of a health event over time is a way to identify long-term (secular) trends. It is useful to note significant events that may have influenced secular trends on graphs of surveillance data. These events may include implementation or cessation of intervention programs, changes in the case definition used for surveillance, changes in public awareness of a condition, or increased intensity of surveillance. In addition, the delay between the occurrence of health outcome and reporting of the problem should be considered when analyzing surveillance data by time. To minimize inaccuracies in the data, the interval between case identification and report must be identified and used consistently for reporting of all cases. Selecting the appropriate interval for analysis is dependent on the health condition under study and can range from time of exposure to expression of symptoms, from symptoms to diagnosis, or from diagnosis to report of case to public health authorities.

Place. Analysis by place can help identify where an increase in cases is occurring and may also reveal isolated outbreaks of a health event that were not detected in the analysis by time. For example, even if the overall numbers of a particular problem are decreasing, levels (including increases) of the number of cases may vary by geographic location. The identification of these focal areas allows prevention resources to be targeted effectively. The size of the unit for geographical analysis is determined by the type of health event under surveillance. For example, for some rare conditions, large areas such as states or countries may be appropriate, whereas for events that occur frequently or for outbreak situations, smaller areas may be more appropriate. However, the use of smaller geographic areas must be balanced with a need for enough data to provide stable estimates. Analysis by place can be carried out using maps or tables; the availability of computers and software for spatial mapping allows more sophisticated analysis of surveillance data by place.

Person. The analysis of surveillance data by person provides information on the characteristics of those experiencing the health problem or those most likely to be exposed to the health event under surveillance. The most frequently used demographic variables for analyses by person are age, gender, and race or ethnicity. Other variables such as marital status, occupation, levels of income, and risk factors for certain health outcomes may be helpful, although most surveillance systems do not routinely collect such information. Surveillance systems have also been used to study behavioral characteristics of populations.

Interactions between time, place, and person can obscure important patterns of disease in specific populations. Proceeding from crude rates to variable-specific rates during the analysis phase may clarify the effects of interactions between time, place, and person and reveal more meaningful trends in the surveillance data. For information on calculating reproductive health rates and ratios using surveillance data, refer to Appendix A.

Framework for Data Analysis

1. Identify appropriate and feasible rates or indicators prior to data collection.
2. Calculate rates, ratios, proportions.
3. Prepare tables, graphs, and charts.
4. Compare rates with expected values, reference rates, and baseline rates.
5. Use statistical probability methods to determine whether apparent differences in rates are significant.
6. Prioritize the most important health problems—cause-specific morbidity and mortality rates.
7. Identify subgroups at highest risk.
8. Identify factors potentially responsible for morbidity and mortality.

Interpretation of Surveillance Data

Adapted from: Janes GR, Hutwagner LC, Cates W Jr, Stroup DF, Williamson GD. Descriptive epidemiology: analyzing and interpreting surveillance data. In: Teutsch SM, Churchill RE, editors. Principles and practice of public health surveillance. 2nd ed. New York: Oxford University Press; 2000. p. 112–67.

Interpretation is the process of transforming the data obtained from the surveillance system into information for action. Quality data play a crucial role in allowing health staff to modify and refine the way they are doing things in the field, and in focusing the attention of policymakers on the health status of a population. Data should not be interpreted in isolation, but rather with a background knowledge of the etiology, epidemiology, and natural history of the disease or health event. Interpretation of surveillance data provides information that can be used in identifying epidemics, monitoring trends, evaluating public policy, and projecting future needs.

Identifying epidemics. Through systematic surveillance, increases of a health event to epidemic proportions can be identified in data analysis. Surveillance data often provide adequate information to detect increases in the prevalence of a health event. In the interpretation phase, it is important to consider whether trends are stable, gradually rise and fall, or show occurrence of an abrupt increase over that which was expected. Several factors, however, could result in an increase in the number of cases reported, including population changes due to migration, improved diagnostic procedures, enhanced reporting techniques, and changes in the surveillance system or methods. Although any variation in the incidence or prevalence of a health event should be taken seriously, it is important to consider these factors when making any inferences.

Monitoring trends. Long-term temporal trends in surveillance data should be explained in the interpretation phase. Surveillance is especially critical in chronic diseases and reproductive health, in which interventions based on long-term trends have more impact than in epidemics, which require rapid investigation and control measures. Collection of regular, systematic surveillance data enables adequate monitoring of various health events and can help in determining appropriate intervention and prevention strategies.

Evaluating public policy. Health interventions and the effect of policies on these interventions can be evaluated using surveillance data. Evaluating surveillance data can enhance management decision-making for more efficient resource utilization, improved program operations, and maximum public benefit.

Projecting future needs. Future trends can be predicted by looking at current surveillance data and applying mathematical models to these data. For example, when changes occur in risk factors among a population at risk for a health event, changes in morbidity and mortality from that health event can be predicted using surveillance data.

Limitations of surveillance data. Several things should be kept in mind when analyzing data from surveillance systems. First, knowledge of the strengths and weaknesses of the data collection methods and reporting system will provide insight on the trends that emerge from the analysis of data; that is, are the observed trends in data "real"? Analysis should proceed from the simplest procedures to the most complex. Be aware of the quality of data collected and of any discrepancies if reporting from multiple sources, because these factors will, in turn, dictate the level of analysis that can be performed on the data with minimum bias and misinterpretation.

The accuracy of surveillance data is evaluated in terms of their *reliability* and *validity*. It is important to know whether the particular health event is reported consistently by different observers (reliability), and also whether reports of the health event under study reflect the true condition as it occurs (validity). Another basic concept to consider in the analysis of surveillance data is ecological fallacy. Ecological fallacy may occur when interpreting observations about groups. Ecological fallacy can be in the form of *aggregation bias*, which arises from loss of information when individuals are grouped, or *specification bias*, which arises from the definition of the group itself. Care should be taken to reduce the chances of ecological fallacy by analyzing subsets of data to reveal disparate trends within the survey data.

Limitations of the collected data must be recognized, interpreted, and reported. Underreporting may be inevitable because most surveillance systems are based on conditions reported by health care providers. However, so long as the underreporting is relatively consistent, incomplete data can still be used to identify disease trends. Another surveillance issue is that reporting biases can distort estimates of disease burden. For example, a health problem that leads to hospitalization may more likely be reported than problems seen on an outpatient basis. This bias may be reduced by adjusting for skewed reporting, or by collecting data from multiple sources where feasible. When interpreting surveillance data, one should be aware of inconsistencies in case definitions and any changes in existing definitions that may affect the accuracy of case reports. Overall, data analysts need to ensure representativeness in the reported cases, consistency in case definitions, and a commitment to enhancing the timeliness in data collection and reporting.

Communication of Findings From Surveillance

Communicating the results of surveillance is the next step in the process of transforming the data into information for action *(22)*. Information generated from surveillance serves to inform and motivate the recipients, so it is more appropriate to *communicate*, rather than simply disseminate, surveillance information. Dissemination implies a one-way process in which information is conveyed from one point to another, whereas communication is a collaborative process involving at least a sender and a recipient. Thus, the process of communicating surveillance data is not complete until recipients acknowledge receipt (dissemination) and comprehension of the information (feedback). Health personnel are more likely to continue the challenging job of collecting information if they know what is being used and acted on.

People who need to receive communication about surveillance information include those who report cases and supply data (e.g., health care providers, laboratory directors), and those who need to know for administrative, program planning, and decision-making purposes *(22)*. It is critical that the results and recommendations generated by the data lead to concrete action for achieving predetermined health objectives. Table 5 lists guidelines for communicating surveillance information:

Table 5. Framework for Disseminating Results of Public Health Surveillance

Controlling and Directing Information Dissemination

Steps	Questions to Be Answered
Establish communications message	What should be said?
Define audience	To whom should it be said?
Select the channel	Through what communication medium?
Market the message	How should the message be stated?
Evaluate the impact	What effect did the message create?

Adapted from: Goodman RA, Remington PL, Howard RJ. Communicating information for action within the public health system. In: Teutsch SM, Churchill RE, editors. Principles and practice of public health surveillance. 2nd ed. New York: Oxford University Press; 2000. p. 168–75.

Depending on available resources and the needs of the audience, many possible channels of communication exist for surveillance data, including simple chalkboards, posters and pamphlets, formal publications, electronic media (telecommunications systems, fax, and audio and videoconferences), mass media, and public forums. Irrespective of the target audience or channel of communication, the information should be presented in a clear and simple format. Graphic formats and other visual displays are likely to be more effective in conveying information than conventional tabular presentations of figures.

The communication aspect of surveillance should be periodically evaluated to ensure that the surveillance information is being communicated to those who need to know and that the information is benefitting the population through initiation of appropriate public health action or response. Although formal evaluations may not always be conducted, these objectives should always be considered when planning the communication of surveillance data. Ultimately, effective communication of public health surveillance information represents the critical link in translating scientific information into public health practice.

Implementing Public Health Action Based on Surveillance Data

The implementation of public health action as a result of information linked through surveillance depends primarily on how effectively the data are disseminated to public health officials and policymakers responsible for directing and funding public health strategies and programs. Analysis and interpretation of surveillance data provide a basis for the identification of problems and possible solutions within the health care sector. Ongoing surveillance activities permit assessment and modification of intervention efforts already in progress. When data are provided in a timely fashion to the health sector, they may be used for the planning, development, implementation, and evaluation of public health programs. This connection between data collection and public health action continues to be the vital link that underscores the value and utility of surveillance as a tool (2).

EVALUATION OF SURVEILLANCE SYSTEMS

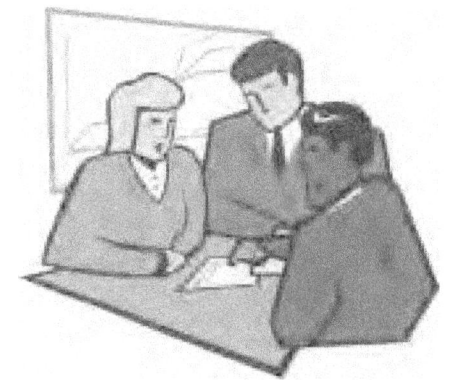

Regular review of an established surveillance system allows health staff to modify and refine health actions taking place in the field. It can also be the first step in assessing how to address the need for surveillance information for a new health outcome—whether that information can be collected by modifying an existing system or whether a new system is needed. Evaluation of surveillance systems is a key step in promoting the best use of public health resources and should include recommendations for improving quality and efficiency. Evaluation of surveillance systems promotes the best use of public health resources by ensuring that public health problems are under surveillance, that surveillance systems operate efficiently, and that information disseminated by surveillance systems is useful for public health practice *(23)*. Evaluation of a public health surveillance system involves an assessment of the system's attributes, including sensitivity, timeliness, representativeness, predictive value, accuracy and completeness of descriptive information, simplicity, flexibility, and acceptability *(23)*. An evaluation of the system must consider those attributes that are of the highest priority for a particular system and its overall objectives.

Elements in Evaluation of Surveillance Systems

A thorough evaluation should identify ways of improving the system's operation and efficiency. CDC has an established system for evaluating surveillance systems *(23)*, which is available at http://www.cdc.gov/mmwr/preview/mmwrhtml/rr5013a1.htm.

Briefly, in evaluating a surveillance system, the following tasks should be conducted:

A. Engage the stakeholder in the evaluation.

B. Describe the surveillance system to be evaluated.

    1. Describe the public health importance of the health-related event under surveillance.

    2. Describe the purpose and operation of the surveillance system.

    3. Describe the resources used to operate the system.

C. Focus the evaluation design.

    1. Determine the specific purpose of the evaluation.

    2. Identify stakeholders who will receive the findings and recommendations of the evaluation.

3. Consider what will be done with the information generated from the evaluation.

4. Specify the questions that will be answered by the evaluation.

5. Determine standards for assessing the performance of the surveillance system.

D. Gather credible evidence regarding the performance of the surveillance system.

1. Indicate the level of usefulness.

2. Describe each system attribute.

E. Justify and state conclusions, making recommendations.

F. Ensure use of evaluation findings and share lessons learned.

CASE STUDY I

AN EVALUATION OF A REPRODUCTIVE HEALTH SURVEILLANCE SYSTEM

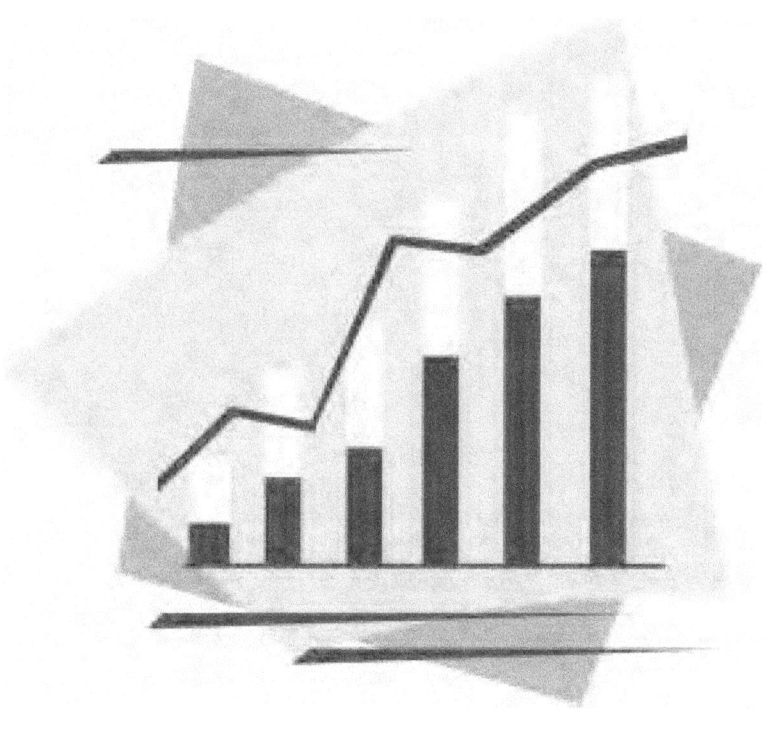

CASE STUDY I: AN EVALUATION OF A REPRODUCTIVE HEALTH SURVEILLANCE SYSTEM

STUDENT VERSION

Learning Objectives

After completing this case study, the participant should be able to:

- Outline the elements of evaluating a surveillance system.

- Discuss the factors contributing to the public health importance of a health event.

- Provide examples of impact, process, and outcome indicators useful in evaluating a reproductive health surveillance system.

- Assess the usefulness of the information being collected and of the information flow of the surveillance system as a whole.

- Evaluate the surveillance system in terms of the following attributes: simplicity, flexibility, acceptability, sensitivity, predictive value positive, representativeness, and timeliness.

CASE STUDY I: AN EVALUATION OF A REPRODUCTIVE HEALTH SURVEILLANCE SYSTEM

Background

The reproductive health of women is especially vulnerable in a crisis situation such as exists at a refugee camp. In addition to the lack of normal sources of reproductive health care (e.g., family planning, prenatal care, safe delivery), the disruption of normal social patterns can lead to sexual violence, unplanned pregnancies, unsafe abortions, and increased incidence of sexually transmitted diseases. Even in the most organized refugee settings, the reproductive health needs of women often go unnoticed and unprotected.

In 1991, Azerbaijan declared its independence from the Soviet Union. In 1992, ethnic Armenians occupied the disputed region of Nagorno-Karabakh and surrounding regions in Azerbaijan. By 1996, there were 845,000 refugees or internally displaced persons (IDPs) in Azerbaijan. The deterioration of the existing health system caused a shift from pregnant women delivering in government hospitals to delivering at home with local midwives instead of government-employed physicians. During this time, there was no effective family planning program in Azerbaijan, mostly due to cultural attitudes, high costs of birth control, and limited availability of and access to up-to-date information.

In 1996, a relief organization established the Reproductive Health Surveillance System to help meet the reproductive health needs of refugee and displaced women in Azerbaijan. By 1998, this organization operated 6 reproductive health clinics and 11 mobile units serving 14 rural districts throughout central Azerbaijan. The following services were offered to the women: a physical, gynecological, and pelvic examination; family planning counseling; STD and PID treatment; reproductive health education; and provision of contraceptive supplies. Abortions were not provided in the clinics; however, women who wished to obtain an abortion were referred to a government hospital. Some of the early findings of the surveillance system showed that a high number of abortions and frequent clinic visits for pelvic infections were occurring among these women. In 1998, an evaluation of this surveillance system was conducted.

Evaluation of Surveillance Systems

Regular review of an established surveillance system allows health staff to modify and refine health actions taking place in the field. Evaluation of surveillance systems is an important step in promoting the best use of public health resources and should include recommendations for improving quality and efficiency. Most importantly, an evaluation should assess whether the system is serving a useful public health function and is meeting the system's objectives.

Q1: Regular review of an established surveillance system is necessary to assess its usefulness, cost, and quality, and to direct possible modifications. List the steps to take in evaluating a surveillance system.

Family Planning, Abortion, and Public Health Burden of PID in Azerbaijan

Abortion has long been the primary method of birth control in Azerbaijan, as in much of the former Soviet Union. According to national statistics, the contraceptive prevalence rate (primarily for oral contraceptive pills and IUDs) was less than 1% before 1992, 1.4% in 1996, and 2% in 1997. The rate of abortions in 1990 was 14 per 100 deliveries. However, after Azerbaijan's independence, the rate of abortions rose to 23 per 100 deliveries in 1994. Alarmingly, data on complications associated with clinical abortions indicate a tremendous increase since the early 1990s.

Data from the Reproductive Health Surveillance System showed that refugee and IDP women visiting clinics were experiencing high rates of postabortion infections, many of which were reported to be pelvic inflammatory disease (PID). Anecdotally, many women were having abortions for "menstrual regulation" without first having a pregnancy test.

PID encompasses a spectrum of inflammatory disorders of the upper female genital tract. It is caused by bacteria, most often those responsible for sexually transmitted diseases such as gonorrhea and chlamydia; other pathogens, such as those that cause bacterial vaginosis, may also be responsible for the development of PID. It is estimated that between 10% and 20% of cervical gonococcal or chlamydial infections may progress to PID when left untreated *(23)*.

Acute PID is difficult to diagnose because of the wide variability in symptoms and severity among women. As a consequence, delay in diagnosis and effective therapy probably contribute to inflammatory sequelae in the upper reproductive tract. Long-term complications of PID include ectopic pregnancy, infertility, pelvic adhesions, and chronic pelvic pain *(24)*. Diagnosis is further complicated by the lack of a widely accepted clinical criteria for PID.

Q2: Health events that affect many people clearly have public health importance, as do events that cluster in time and place, affecting relatively few people. In a refugee setting, reproductive health may not be prioritized until the initial emergency phase is stabilized. However, once high mortality rates are under control and basic needs properly addressed, complete and integrated reproductive health services can be planned *(25)*. What questions would be useful to ask in ascertaining the public health importance of surveillance for PID among refugee women in Azerbaijan?

Evaluation of the Surveillance System for PID

The Reproductive Health Surveillance System had been in place for more than two years before the preliminary evaluation conducted in July 1998. Routine monthly data collected at the stationary clinics indicated that a large proportion of the women had symptoms associated with postabortion pelvic infection, which was considered to be PID. This review of the data helped to define a new program objective to decrease the incidence of symptomatic cases of PID by 15%. In addition, the majority of these symptoms were associated with recent induced abortion. Strategies to reduce the number of PID cases focused on ways to prevent PID associated with induced abortion, including decreasing the number of women relying on abortion as their sole method of birth control and increasing access to family planning services.

The evaluation of surveillance systems generally involves the definition of indicators to track the progress toward explicit, quantifiable, and time-limited objectives *(26)*. Once the objectives of a surveillance system have been defined, indicators are used as markers of progress toward improved reproductive health. Indicators can either be direct measures of impact, or indirect measures of progress toward specified process goals. An indicator can be thought of as a measurement that provides information regarding a health outcome, when compared with a standard or desired level of achievement. Indicators are repeated over time to track progress toward the system objectives. *Impact* indicators provide information on the end result, but do not provide insight into how the outcome was achieved. For this reason, combining impact indicators with *process* (program activities) and *outcome* (results of those activities) indicators provides the best information to evaluate a surveillance system.

Q3: What is the new program objective adopted after the preliminary evaluation in July 1998?

Q4: In terms of the surveillance system for PID among Azeri refugee women, fill in the blank spaces below with examples of each of the three indicators that could be used to track progress toward achieving the objectives of the system.

Useful Indicators for Evaluating a Reproductive Health Surveillance System

Type	Description	Reproductive Health Example
Impact	Reflects changes in health status expected to result from program activities	
Outcome	Reflects changes in knowledge, attitudes, behaviors, or the availability of necessary services that result from program activities	
Process	Specifies the actions needed for program implementation in order to achieve the intended impact and outcomes	

Once the indicators are in place, it may be necessary to restructure the surveillance system to collect information relevant to the indicator. An assessment of the monthly surveillance form in use before the evaluation revealed several missing links between program objectives and data being collected in the field. It was found that the information being collected was inadequate for determining the differences in incidence of postabortion-complicated and nonprocedure-related cases of symptomatic PID. Data on the hospital performing the abortion were not being collected. There were no data collected on IUD insertion and incidence of PID. Also, self-reported PID was not being captured. However, after the addition of a few simple questions that served to distinguish between the causes of infection, health workers would be able to evaluate trends in PID visits, estimate the proportion of PID likely due to postabortion complications, and examine the impact of health education and interventions on PID prevention. In this way, the surveillance system became linked to the program objective of reducing the incidence of symptomatic cases of PID by 15%.

Once the collection of relevant surveillance data has begun, simple calculations may be useful in monitoring monthly progress. Monthly reporting can be used as a way of showing what work is being done in the field, as well as producing a measurable improvement in the indicators. The following is an example of a simple chart that could be included in monthly feedback reports:

Number of Postabortion-Complicated Cases of PID, August–September 1998

	August 1998	September 1998
Number of postabortion infection cases seen in clinics	195	188
Number of women diagnosed with postabortion-complicated PID	177	145
Percentage of postabortion-complicated PID cases out of total number of postabortion infection cases	90%	77%

In August and September of 1998, a large proportion of women classified as "postabortion infectional" was diagnosed with postabortion-complicated PID, providing strong evidence for the relationship between abortion and PID. Perhaps the most effective way of presenting this information is *graphically*, so that anyone can see at a glance the trend from month to month. When presented graphically, for instance, as a line graph of the percentage of PID cases out of total number of postabortion infectional cases seen each month, the information could be used as a tool to focus the attention of decision makers on PID as a public health problem, mobilize public health resources to address PID treatment and prevention, and guide and refine the relief program that is being put in place. In sum, "good" data are reliable, accurate, and presented in a way that anyone can understand *(16)*.

Q5: Develop a shell of a graph to monitor whether the new program objective is being met, based on the indicators. Label the axes, title, and key of the graph.

Case Definition of PID

In this refugee setting, women attending any of the six stationary reproductive health clinics present potentially important opportunities for the detection and management of PID. Despite comprehensive physical examinations, many episodes of PID go unrecognized. Although some cases are asymptomatic, others are undiagnosed because of mild or nonspecific symptoms. Without a clear case definition, it is also possible that some cases of "postabortion infection" may have been diagnosed as PID erroneously. The lack of sensitive, specific, rapid, and inexpensive diagnostic tests for PID is a significant obstacle for case ascertainment, particularly among asymptomatic women.

The wide variability of PID symptoms necessitates an alternative strategy for clinical diagnosis. In detecting symptomatic cases of PID, the use of clinical algorithms based on risk assessment and symptoms is an alternative strategy in settings with limited access to diagnostic tests. This strategy, also known as the *syndromic approach*, requires experience and continued training of clinicians and can significantly influence the yield of case ascertainment. Using this approach, a case of PID is identified if all of the following minimum criteria are present: 1) lower abdominal tenderness and pain; 2) adnexal tenderness; and 3) cervical motion tenderness. Additional criteria used to support a diagnosis of PID are oral temperature over 101°F and abnormal cervical or vaginal discharge *(27)*. This case definition was adopted by the clinics, and health care providers were quickly trained in the use of the syndromic approach.

Q6: What is the case definition of PID for this surveillance system? Assess the ability of the surveillance system to capture symptomatic cases of PID.

The target population for PID surveillance is women attending any one of six stationary reproductive health clinics in Azerbaijan. The doctor or midwife for every woman seen at the stationary clinics fills out the women's health card and the Women's Reproductive Health (WRH) register each day. The data from the cards are tallied and entered on daily reporting forms. Each week, the daily reporting forms are compiled and sent to Baku, the capital city.

Information generated from surveillance serves to inform and motivate the recipients, thereby enhancing collaboration and improving the level of reporting to the system. The surveillance report should include summary information on the occurrence of the health event by person, place, and time. In the surveillance system for PID, a data specialist computerizes and compiles a morbidity and mortality monthly report using the daily reporting forms. This report is generated within one week of the end of each month and disseminated for trend analysis and program development. The quarterly report is compiled and written by the field coordinator, and reviewed by the medical coordinator and country director in Baku. In order to provide information for appropriate action by health workers and decision makers, the quarterly report is disseminated to the relief organizations headquarters in the United States, the donor (United Nations High Commission on Refugees), and the Ministry of Health in Baku.

Q7: Is the Reproductive Health Surveillance System a population-based or facility-based system? What are the advantages and disadvantages of this type of system? How might the type of system affect the reported prevalence of PID in this population?

Often it is useful to sketch a simple flowchart to better illustrate the steps involved in processing the data obtained through the surveillance system. This chart can help to answer the following important questions:

- What information is being collected? Is it what programs need?

- What are the reporting sources? Who is supposed to report? Who actually does report?

- How are the data handled? How are they routed, transferred, and stored? Are there unnecessary delays?

- How are the data analyzed? By whom? How often?

- How is the information disseminated? How often are reports distributed? To whom? Is the information getting to all those who need to know?

Q8: Draw a simple sketch of the existing flow of data, and suggest some changes that would enhance the ability of those using the data to make decisions and take actions.

It is important to give feedback to the workers in the field who are the primary source of information. Discussions with clinic health workers revealed that they found the data collection system acceptable and not too burdensome; however, they felt that they were not receiving any feedback. For this reason, it is suggested that a link between the office in Baku and the local clinic staff would strengthen the surveillance system. This linkage, indicated by the dotted line (page 57), should enhance the timeliness of the system by making data available to local clinic staff both for immediate control efforts and for long-term program planning. At all levels of the system, the analyzed data should be used to reassess system indicators and to confirm whether program objectives have been met.

Action

The recommendations from the July 1998 evaluation of the Reproductive Health Surveillance System included the following:

- Change in objectives to focus on an important reproductive health problem in this population.

- Change in indicators to monitor progress toward this objective.

- Change in data forms to collect information to calculate the indicators.

- Change in case definition for PID and training in how to use this case definition.

Most of these changes were instituted during the following month, and the statistics for August and September 1998 reflected these changes. The health care providers quickly adapted to the new forms and were enthusiastic about their training in the syndromic approach in order to use the new PID case definition. With appropriate training and information, clinic health staff were able to adjust to using the syndromic approach to PID case detection with little difficulty.

Below are some data from the August and September 1998 monthly reporting forms.

	August 1998	September 1998
Number of sexually active women seen in the clinics	1,123	987
Postabortion infectional	195	188
PID Postabortion	177	145
Not abortion-related	1	7
Number of women using contraception	512	460

Q9: What indicators can you calculate from the table above? What are the interpretations of these indicators and the data from the table?

In addition to the actions taken to modify the surveillance system and change clinical practice, the results from the Reproductive Health Surveillance System were used to develop a retrospective cohort study to test the hypothesis that women who undergo abortions are at increased risk of PID. Preliminary results from this study show that although abortion itself is not associated with PID, the following risk factors are:

- Husband or partner with a sexually transmitted infection.
- No antibiotics during the last abortion.
- Abortion without confirming pregnancy with a pregnancy test first.
- Preexisting bacterial vaginosis infection (although chlamydia and gonorrhea infection were not associated with PID).

Because of the low number of women using methods of contraception in this population, the relief organization has worked with other relief agencies in Azerbaijan as well as the Ministry of Health, to increase family planning services and supplies at the national level for refugees/IDPs as well as for the general population.

Cost

The yearly budget for the operation of the reproductive health program was $140,000 in 1997. This amount covers both the clinical care and the surveillance components of the six reproductive health clinics, including salaries, clinic equipment, travel and transportation, printing, and publishing reports.

Attributes of the PID Surveillance System in Azerbaijan

Several qualities or attributes affect the operation and usefulness of a surveillance system. The *simplicity* of a surveillance system refers both to its structure and ease of operation. Ideally, a surveillance system should be as simple as possible, while still meeting its objectives. The *flexibility* of a system is defined as the ability of a system to adapt to changing needs or operating conditions with little additional time, personnel, or allocated funds. In general, simpler systems will be more flexible since fewer components will need to be modified when adapting the system. The flexibility of a system often is judged best retrospectively, after a change has been put in place and its impact on the system can be evaluated. The *acceptability* of a system reflects the willingness of individuals and organizations to participate in the surveillance system.

The primary means of assessing the *sensitivity* of a surveillance system is to estimate the proportion of the total number of cases in the population being detected by the system, assuming that most reported cases are correctly classified. The sensitivity of a surveillance system is affected by the likelihood that 1) persons with the health condition will seek medical care; 2) the disease will be diagnosed, reflecting the skill of health care workers and the sensitivity of diagnostic tests; and 3) given the diagnosis, the case will be reported to the system. Increasing the sensitivity of a system may enhance the detection of epidemics and the understanding of the natural course of an adverse health event in a defined population. With respect to surveillance, *predictive value positive* (PVP) is defined as the proportion of persons identified as cases who actually have the health event under surveillance. The PVP is directly related to the sensitivity and specificity of the health event, as well as the prevalence of the condition in the population; the PVP increases with increasing specificity and prevalence. A *representative* surveillance system accurately characterizes the epidemiologic characteristics of a health event in a defined population and time frame. *Timeliness* refers to the availability of data and information in time for appropriate action and reflects the speed or delay between steps in a surveillance system. Improving the timeliness of a surveillance system allows control and prevention activities to be initiated earlier.

Q10: Discuss the surveillance system for PID with respect to the following attributes: simplicity, flexibility, acceptability, sensitivity, predictive value positive, representativeness, and timeliness.

Q11: Describe the usefulness of this surveillance system. What have the data from this surveillance system been used for and what impact has the system had on reproductive health care for refugees in Azerbaijan?

Answers

Q1: Regular review of an established surveillance system is necessary to assess its usefulness, cost, and quality, and to direct possible modifications. List the steps to take in evaluating a surveillance system.

A1:

a) Describe the public health importance of the health event.

b) Describe the surveillance system to be evaluated.

- List the objectives of the system.
- Describe the health system under surveillance, including the case definition.
- Draw a flowchart or diagram of the system.
- Describe the components and operation of the system.

Include information on surveillance population, time frame of data collection, type of information collected, transfer and analysis of data, and distribution of reports.

c) Assess the level of usefulness of the surveillance system by describing actions taken as a result of the data generated by the system.

d) Evaluate the system in terms of the following attributes:

Simplicity – the extent to which a surveillance system is uncomplicated in structure and easy to operate.

Flexibility – the extent to which a surveillance system can adapt to changing information needs or operating conditions with little additional cost.

Acceptability – the willingness of individuals and organizations to participate in the surveillance system.

Sensitivity – an estimate of the proportion of the total number of cases in the community being detected by the system.

Predictive Value Positive (PVP) – the proportion of persons identified as cases who actually have the condition under surveillance.

Representativeness – the extent to which the surveillance system accurately characterizes the epidemiologic characteristics of a health event in a defined population.

Timeliness – the speed or delay between steps in the surveillance system.

e) Compare the direct costs of operating the surveillance system with the benefits obtained.

f) List your recommendations, addressing whether the system is meeting its objectives.

Q2: Health events that affect many people clearly have public health importance, as do events that cluster in time and place, affecting relatively few people. In a refugee setting, reproductive health may not be prioritized until the initial emergency phase is stabilized. However, once high mortality rates are under control and basic needs properly addressed, complete and integrated reproductive health services can be planned *(26)*. What questions would be useful to ask in ascertaining the public health importance of surveillance for PID among refugee women in Azerbaijan?

A2:
a) What are some measures of burden of disease, for example, total number of cases, incidence, prevalence of PID among refugee/internally displaced women in Azerbaijan, number of postabortion-complicated cases of PID, number of symptomatic cases of PID associated with IUD insertion, number of referrals for abortions?

b) Is an identifiable subgroup of the population at greater risk for PID, for example, women with histories of abortion, women referred to particular hospitals for abortions, women of certain age groups, women with histories of IUD insertion?

c) Are there efficacious treatments or preventive measures for PID? And, furthermore, what are the physical, social, and emotional sequelae of undetected and/or untreated PID?

d) What are the direct and indirect costs associated with PID, for example, medical-care expenses and lost worktime?

Q3: What is the new program objective adopted after the preliminary evaluation in July 1998?

A3: Decrease the incidence of symptomatic cases of PID by 15%.

Q4: In terms of the surveillance system for PID among Azeri refugee women, fill in the blank spaces below with examples of each of the three indicators that could be used to track progress toward achieving the objectives of the system.

A4: In keeping with the objective of decreasing the incidence of symptomatic PID by 15%, an example of an impact indicator is the

Useful Indicators for Evaluating a Reproductive Health Surveillance System

Type	Description	Reproductive Health Example
Impact	Reflects changes in health status expected to result from program activities	Percentage of women with postabortion-complicated cases of PID
Outcome	Reflects changes in knowledge, attitudes, behaviors, or the availability of necessary services that result from program activities	Percentage of women relying on abortion as their sole method of birth control
Process	Specifies the actions needed for program implementation in order to achieve the intended impact and outcomes	Percentage of clinic providers trained in family planning services

percentage of women with postabortion-complicated cases of PID seen at the clinics each month. Outcome indicators relate directly to the priority intervention, the target population, or those charged with caring for the target population. The percentage of women relying on abortion as their sole method of birth control is an example of an outcome indicator that you would expect to decrease with the intervention. Process indicators correspond to various activities necessary to achieve the intended outcomes and impact, for example, training, supply of drugs and equipment, and health education. In this refugee setting, the percentage of health workers trained in providing family planning services could be used as a process indicator.

Q5: Develop a shell of a graph to monitor whether the new program objective is being met, based on the indicators. Label the axes, title, and key of the graph.

A5: This is one example of a shell of a graph to monitor the indicators.

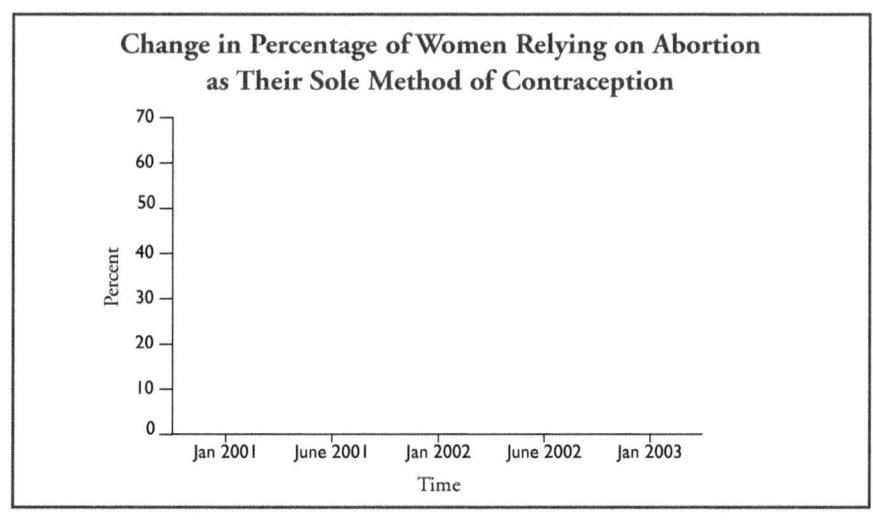

Q6: What is the case definition of PID for this surveillance system? Assess the ability of the surveillance system to capture symptomatic cases of PID.

A6: A case of PID is identified if all of the following minimum criteria are present: 1) lower abdominal tenderness and pain; 2) adnexal tenderness; and 3) cervical motion tenderness. Additional criteria used to support a diagnosis of PID are oral temperature over 101°F and abnormal cervical or vaginal discharge.

In the clinics, the sensitivity of the system in detecting true cases of PID among refugee women is judged to be poor, mainly due to imprecise syndrome diagnosis, the lack of a gold standard, and the variability in clinical presentation. It is thought that a meaningful proportion of true cases of PID are not being captured by the system. As health workers become better trained in using the syndromic approach to PID detection, the proportion of true cases to the total number of cases classified as PID should increase.

Q7: Is the Reproductive Health Surveillance System a population-based or facility-based system? What are the advantages and disadvantages of this type of system? How might the type of system affect the reported prevalence of PID in this population?

A7: The Reproductive Health System is a facility-based system. Advantages of this system include a relatively simple method of data collection in a defined facility-based population, with clinical verification of diagnoses and follow-up. The main disadvantage is the lack of information about women with PID who do not come to the clinic. This situation may cause the prevalence of PID to be severely underestimated especially because PID is often asymptomatic and women may not come to the clinic for treatment.

Q8: Draw a simple sketch of the existing flow of data, and suggest some changes that would enhance the ability of those using the data to make decisions and take actions.

A8:

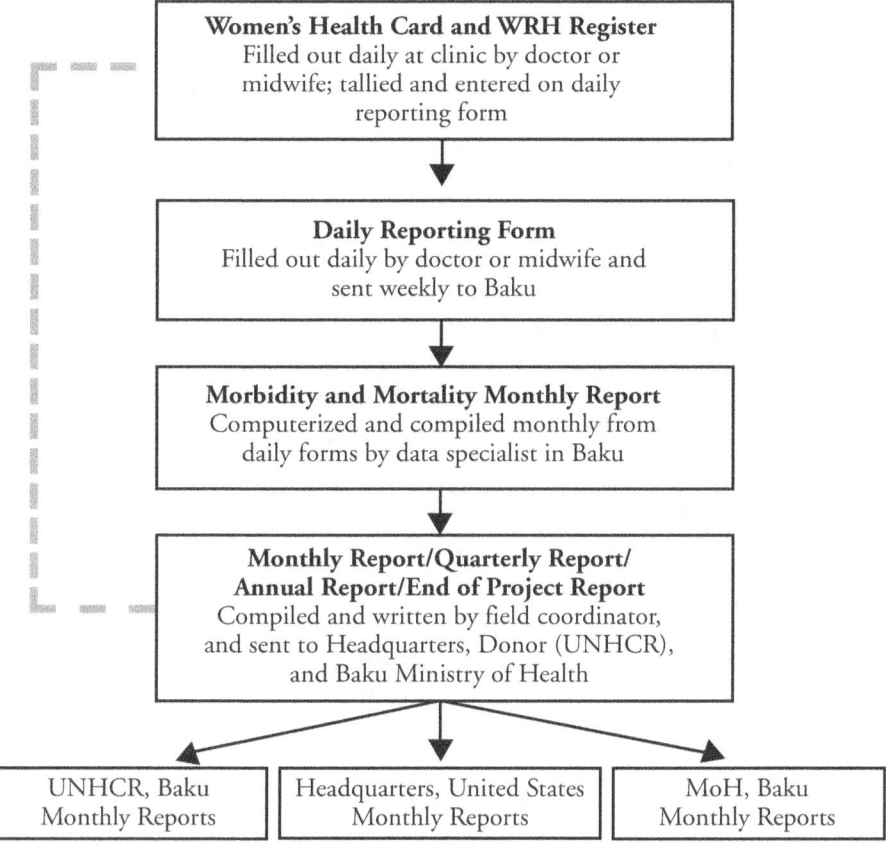

Q9: What indicators can you calculate from the table below? What are the interpretations of these indicators and the data from the table?

A9:

a) Indicators:

	August 1998	September 1998
Percentage of women in clinics with PID	177/1,123 = 15.8%	145/987 = 14.7%
Percentage of PID cases associated with abortion	177/178 = 99.4%	145/152 = 95.4%
Percentage of women using a family planning method	512/1,123 = 45.6%	460/987 = 46.6%

b) Interpretation:
The prevalence of PID among women seen at RI clinics is about 15% (magnitude of problem). In these 2 months, the vast majority of PID is occurring among women who have had recent abortions (group at high risk). About 40%–45% of women are using family planning; therefore, a large percentage of women may be relying on abortion as their primary means of family planning.

Q10: Discuss the surveillance system for PID with respect to the following attributes: simplicity, flexibility, acceptability, sensitivity, predictive value positive, representativeness, and timeliness.

A10: The surveillance system for PID is judged to be relatively simple, due to minimal levels and complexity of reporting. The information being collected on PID is extremely simple, to the point that additional questions are needed in order to calculate the indicators to judge whether the system is meeting the program objectives.

The system has proven to be sufficiently flexible in accommodating the changes in program priorities. In spite of changes made to the surveillance forms, data compilation and reporting are accomplished in a timely fashion. With appropriate training and information, clinic health staff were able to adjust to using the syndromic approach to PID case detection with little difficulty.

PID surveillance among refugee women is acceptable, since PID has been recognized as a major public health issue in this setting. An assessment of the daily forms and monthly surveillance forms reveals that health workers are collecting complete information.

The sensitivity of the PID surveillance system would be assessed by estimating the proportion of the total number of refugee women who truly have PID that were captured by the system. The sensitivity of the system is judged to be poor, mostly because of the variability in clinical presentation and resulting imprecise syndrome diagnosis, as well as the unavailability of gold standard diagnostic tests. Furthermore, doctors and midwives require information and training in order to properly apply the syndromic approach to PID detection.

In this setting, the PVP is defined as the proportion of refugee women diagnosed as having PID who truly have the condition. As the PVP is closely related to the clarity and specificity of the case definition, the PVP in detecting true cases of PID is judged to be poor.

Any selection bias introduced into the surveillance system has the effect of decreasing its representativeness; therefore, significant subpopulations excluded by the system must be identified. The integration of data collection in the 11 mobile reproductive health units operating in 14 rural districts throughout the central region of the country would add to the representativeness of the data generated by the surveillance system.

Even after the modifications to the data collection forms, the first two monthly summary reports were finalized and disseminated to the key players in the health system at the regular schedule, within one week of the end of the previous month. Hence this system would be judged to be timely, since the short interval between data collection and analysis allows for early detection of trends in PID occurrence.

Q11: Describe the usefulness of this surveillance system. What have the data from this surveillance system been used for and what impact has the system had on reproductive health care for refugees in Azerbaijan?

A11:

a) Magnitude of problem: the surveillance system has collected information to estimate the magnitude of PID and abortion-related PID in refugee/IDP women visiting the clinics.

b) Identification of high-risk groups: because the vast majority of women with PID had recently had an abortion, it was hypothesized that abortions were a major cause of PID in this population.

c) Generate hypotheses and stimulate research: based on the above hypothesis, a retrospective cohort study was undertaken to test the hypothesis that induced abortion was a risk factor for PID in this population.

d) Prioritize public health services: because of the high number of abortions, the high rate of abortion-associated PID, and the low contraceptive prevalence in this population, the relief organization is working with other relief organizations and the Ministry of Health to increase family planning services and supplies for all women in Azerbaijan.

CASE STUDY II

AN EVALUATION OF THE PERINATAL SURVEILLANCE SYSTEM OF THE HOST COUNTRY

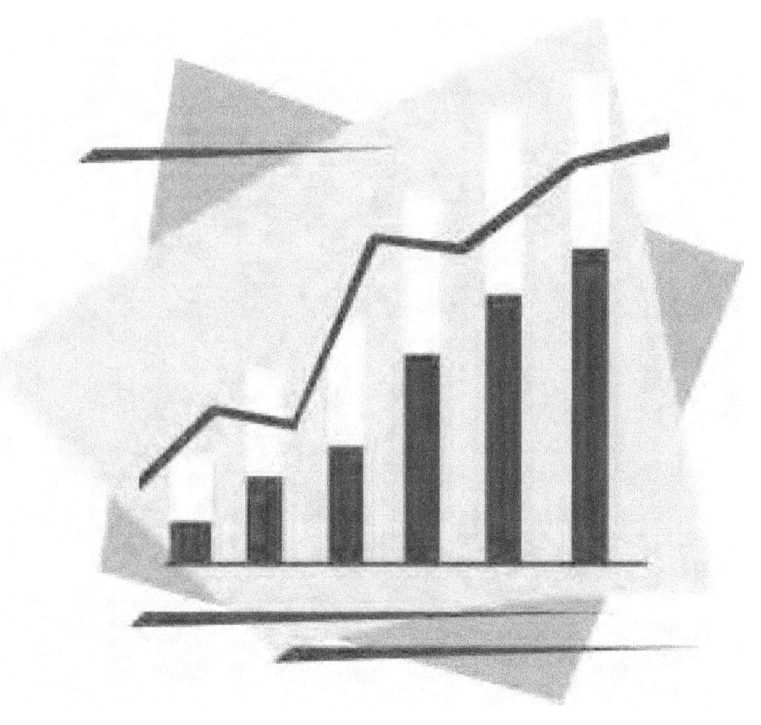

CASE STUDY II: AN EVALUATION OF THE PERINATAL SURVEILLANCE SYSTEM OF THE HOST COUNTRY

Learning Objectives

After completing this case study, the participant should be able to:

- Describe a perinatal (or other) surveillance system, specific to the host country.

- Outline the elements of evaluating a surveillance system.

- Discuss the factors contributing to the public health importance of a health event.

- Provide examples of process and outcome indicators useful in evaluating a reproductive health surveillance system.

- Assess the usefulness of the information being collected and of the information flow of the surveillance system as a whole.

- Evaluate the surveillance system in terms of the following attributes: simplicity, flexibility, acceptability, sensitivity, predictive value positive, representativeness, and timeliness.

- Make recommendations for modifying the current perinatal surveillance system in the host country.

CASE STUDY II: AN EVALUATION OF THE PERINATAL SURVEILLANCE SYSTEM OF THE HOST COUNTRY

Note to Instructors

This case study is meant to familiarize students with current data collection systems in their country and to allow students to evaluate and adapt the current system to meet their goals and objectives for perinatal surveillance. Although this exercise focuses on perinatal outcomes, this process could be easily adapted to focus on another health outcome of interest to students. Questions in this case study may also need to be slightly modified, depending on the level of surveillance information currently available in the country. For example, in countries with no formal perinatal surveillance system in existence, students will focus more on developing a system to meet their needs. In countries with more established systems, students will focus more on evaluating the current system and making recommendations.

Materials needed: Before the case study, the instructor will need to gather the relevant vital statistics and other forms currently in use in the country, as well as a description of the vital statistics system. You may want to ask a few students to do this in advance.

Students should break into teams of four to five participants.

AN EVALUATION OF THE PERINATAL SURVEILLANCE SYSTEM OF THE HOST COUNTRY

Background

You are a member of your country's Task Force on Perinatal Surveillance charged with evaluating current information systems regarding perinatal health and making recommendations for any changes to improve surveillance of perinatal health.

Q1: A successful task force for evaluating a surveillance system is made up of stakeholders, who will be involved in planning, implementing, and using the findings of the surveillance system and its evaluation. Stakeholders may include members of the local, regional, and national levels of the Ministry of Health, other government and community leaders, public health practitioners, health care providers, maternal and child health programmers, members of the community, and professional and voluntary organizations. Decide who the stakeholders for a perinatal surveillance system in your country are, and decide who in your team will represent each stakeholder.

Goals and Objectives of the Perinatal Surveillance System

The first step in either developing or evaluating a surveillance system is to identify the goals and objectives of the surveillance system. These goals and objectives are generally closely tied to the programmatic goals and objectives, which are monitored by the surveillance system. For example, a programmatic goal may be to reduce perinatal mortality due to obstructed labor, with the specific objective of increasing the proportion of births by cesarean section. This example leads to a surveillance system goal of being able to monitor perinatal mortality, with three specific measurement objectives: 1) perinatal mortality, 2) cause of perinatal mortality, and 3) mode of delivery.

Q2: What are your goals and objectives for your Perinatal Surveillance System? How do these relate to programmatic goals and objectives?

Once you have clearly defined goals and objectives, you are ready to identify the indicators you will need, and, therefore, the data elements necessary for your surveillance system.

Q3: For five priority objectives, list the appropriate indicators, type of indicator, definition, and specific data source, using the following table. You may not be able to list data sources for all of your indicators—this will allow you to see what data are currently available to you and what data you may need to collect.

Objective	Indicator	Type of Indicator (process, outcome)	Definition	Data Source
Example: To measure mode of delivery	C-section rate	Process	Number of pregnant women with C-section in a specific time and geographic period Number of deliveries in the same time period and geographic area	Form #1201 – Hospital delivery log Vital statistics

After you have filled in the table, discuss the following questions:

a) What is your balance of process versus outcome indicators? If you have more process indicators than outcome indicators, you may need to re-evaluate your priorities. Are these priority indicators really going to allow you to assess your overall goal?

b) Are there indicators for which you do not have a data source? If so, discuss the trade-offs between creating a new data element for the surveillance system versus dropping the indicator.

Describing and Evaluating the Perinatal Surveillance System

Now that you have established goals, objectives, and indicators, and the task force has a clear idea of what it wants to accomplish, it is time to describe the surveillance system that will help you meet your objectives. The next steps will largely depend on your country's current surveillance system. If you have a fairly well-developed perinatal surveillance system in place, you will want to focus on evaluating and modifying the current system to meet your needs. If your country does not have a perinatal system in place, you will want to focus on developing that system, incorporating as many of the current data collection systems as possible (e.g., vital statistics, health facility reporting).

Q4: Refer to Appendix C. Updated Guidelines for Evaluating Public Health Surveillance Systems *(28)*.

a) Describe the public health importance of perinatal health issues in your country (i.e., why do you need a perinatal surveillance system).

b) Describe the components of the perinatal surveillance system:

- Data collection

- Data analysis

- Interpretation

- Communication and dissemination

- Action

c) Draw a flowchart of the perinatal surveillance system.

d) Using the current data collection forms, are you able to collect the necessary data for the indicators? If not, is the indicator important enough to collect a new data element? If so, how will that data element be collected?

Q5: Evaluate the perinatal surveillance system, including its usefulness, attributes, and cost (refer to Appendix C. Updated Guidelines for Evaluating Public Health Surveillance Systems).

Q6: What are the recommendations the task force will make to the Ministry of Health for modifying the current surveillance system or designing a new one?

APPENDIX A.

COMMONLY USED RATES IN REPRODUCTIVE HEALTH EPIDEMIOLOGY

APPENDIX A. COMMONLY USED RATES IN REPRODUCTIVE HEALTH EPIDEMIOLOGY

Several epidemiologic measures can be used in reproductive health surveillance as indicators of process and outcome. Please see individual chapters for detailed descriptions of definitions, uses, and interpretations of topic-specific measures. The following is a list of some of the most commonly used measures:

Rate or Ratio	Indicator of	Type of Indicator	Calculation	
Maternal mortality ratio (MMR)	Risk of death due to pregnancy	Impact	$$\frac{\text{Number of maternal deaths occurring in a given time period}}{\text{Number of live births in the same time period}}$$	x 100,000
Maternal mortality rate	Risk of death due to pregnancy	Impact	$$\frac{\text{Number of maternal deaths occurring in a given time period}}{\text{Number of women of reproductive age}}$$	x 1,000
Proportionate mortality	Percentage of deaths due to pregnancy	Impact	$$\frac{\text{Number of maternal deaths in a given time period}}{\text{Number of deaths to women of reproductive age in same time period}}$$	x 100
Cause-specific proportionate mortality	Percentage of maternal deaths due to specific cause	Impact	$$\frac{\text{Number of maternal deaths due to a specific cause}}{\text{Total number of maternal deaths due to all causes}}$$	x 100
Antenatal care coverage	Coverage of antenatal care	Outcome	$$\frac{\text{Number of pregnant women who are attended at least once by trained personnel and who deliver in the specified time period}}{\text{Number of live births in the specified time period}}$$	
Infant vaccination coverage	Coverage of infant vaccination	Outcome	$$\frac{\text{Number of children aged 12–23 months who were fully vaccinated before their first birthday}}{\text{Number of children aged 12–23 months}}$$	
Perinatal mortality rate	Deaths during the perinatal period	Impact	$$\frac{\text{Number of deaths during the perinatal period (from 22 weeks gestation through 7 days of life), or other specified time period}}{\text{Total number of births (live births plus fetal deaths) during the same time period}}$$	x 1,000

continued

Rate or Ratio	Indicator of	Type of Indicator	Calculation
Neonatal mortality rate	Deaths of live infants during the neonatal period	Impact	$\dfrac{\text{Number of live-born infants who die within} < 28 \text{ days in the specified time period}}{\text{Number of live births in the same time period}} \times 1{,}000$
Low birth weight percentage	Number of live-born infants weighing < 2,500 grams	Impact	$\dfrac{\text{Number of live-born infants weighing} < 2{,}500 \text{ grams in the specified time period}}{\text{Total number of live births (birth weight recorded) in the same time period}} \times 100$
STD incidence rate	Incidence of STDs	Impact	$\dfrac{\text{Number of new cases of STDs reported in a specified time period}}{\text{Total population}} \times 1{,}000$
STD prevalence rate (among women who deliver)	Prevalence of STDs among pregnant women	Impact	$\dfrac{\text{Number of women who deliver in the specified time period that test positive for a particular STD}}{\text{Number of women who deliver in the same time period who were tested for that STD}}$
Stillbirth rate	Number of infants born dead	Impact	$\dfrac{\text{Number of infants} > 21 \text{ weeks/500 grams born dead in the specified time period}}{\text{Total number of live births and stillbirths in the same time period}}$
Referral rate	Proportion of women with potential or actual obstetric complications moving from one level of care to another	Outcome	$\dfrac{\text{Number of women with a potential or actual obstetric complication moved to another site}}{\text{Total number of women with obstetric complications in the same area and within the same time period}}$
Cesarean section rate	Proportion of women who have a cesarean section in a specific geographic area in a given time period	Outcome	$\dfrac{\text{Number of live-born infants delivered by cesarean section in a specific time and geographic area}}{\text{Number of live births in the same geographic area and time period}}$

APPENDIX B.

REPRODUCTIVE HEALTH REFERENCE RATES AND RATIOS

APPENDIX B. REPRODUCTIVE HEALTH REFERENCE RATES AND RATIOS

Adapted from: Reproductive health in refugee settings: an inter-agency field manual.
Geneva, Switzerland: United Nations High Commissioner for Refugees; 1999. p. 110.

The following figures have been collected from various sources and cover different time periods. They are intended to give estimates of what may be expected in some populations. These figures indicate a possible range and may assist with resource planning and targeting specific programs—they are **not** intended to be used as definitive baseline rates or as rates to be achieved.

Abortions	10%–15%	of all pregnancies may spontaneously abort before 20 weeks gestation
	90%	of these will occur during the first 3 months
	15%–20%	of all spontaneous abortions that occur require medical interventions
Hypertensive Disorder of Pregnancy (HDP) or Pre-eclampsia	5%–20%	of all pregnancies will develop HDP
	5%–25%	of all primigravida pregnancies will develop HDP
Labor and Delivery Complications	15%	of all pregnancies will require some type of intervention at delivery
	3%–7%	of all pregnancies will require a cesarean section
	10%–15%	of all women will have some degree of cephalopelvic disproportion (higher in poorer socioeconomic populations)
	10%	of deliveries will involve a secondary postpartum hemorrhage (within 24 hours of delivery)
	0.1%–1.0%	of deliveries will involve a secondary postpartum hemorrhage (occurring 24 hours or more after delivery)
	0.1%–0.4%	deliveries will result in uterine rupture
	0.25%–2.4%	of all deliveries will result in some type of birth trauma to the baby
	1.5%	of all births will have a congenital malformation (does not include cardiac malformations diagnosed later in neonatal period)
	31%	of these malformations will result in death

Reference Rates and Ratios for Reproductive Health Indicators

Regional Indicators			
Indicator	**Sub-Saharan Africa**	**Southeast Asia and Pacific**	**Industrialized Countries**
Safe Motherhood			
Crude Birth Rate (per 1,000 population) 44		26	13
Neonatal Mortality Rate (per 1,000 live births) 53		36	5
Perinatal Mortality Rate (per 1,000 live births) 83		51	8
Maternal Mortality Ratio (per 100,000 live births) 971		447	31
Infant Mortality Rate (per 1,000 live births) 97		50	14
Coverage of Antenatal Care (%) 63		65	95
Low Birth Weight Percentage (per 100 live births) 16		15	6
Births attended by trained health personnel (%) 42		53	99
Institutional Deliveries (% of live births) 20		41	98
Unsafe Abortion (1,000 women 15–49) 26		15	1
Anemia in Pregnant Women (%) 52		57	18
Coverage of Tetanus Vaccination (Pregnant Women) 46		49	—
STDs, including HIV/AIDS			
STD Incidence Rate (per 1,000 population) 254		160	77
AIDS Cases (per 100,000) 94		80	27
Family Planning			
Contraceptive Prevalence Rate 15.9		53.2	70.5

Source: United Nations Development Programme. Human Development Report. New York: United Nations; 1997. World Health Organization. World Health Report. Geneva, Switzerland: World Health Organization; 1996. (Adapted from: Reproductive health in refugee settings: an inter-agency field manual. Geneva, Switzerland: United Nations High Commissioner for Refugees; 1999. p. 111.)

APPENDIX C.

UPDATED GUIDELINES FOR EVALUATING PUBLIC HEALTH SURVEILLANCE SYSTEMS

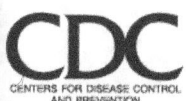

July 27, 2001 / Vol. 50 / No. RR-13

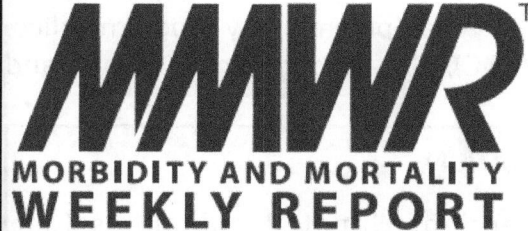

MORBIDITY AND MORTALITY WEEKLY REPORT

Recommendations and Reports

Inside: Continuing Education Examination

Updated Guidelines for Evaluating Public Health Surveillance Systems

Recommendations from the Guidelines Working Group

U.S. DEPARTMENT OF HEALTH AND HUMAN SERVICES
Centers for Disease Control and Prevention (CDC)
Atlanta, GA 30333

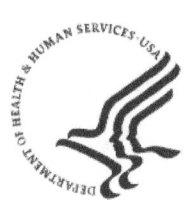

he *MMWR* series of publications is published by the Epidemiology Program Office, Centers for Disease Control and Prevention (CDC), U.S. Department of Health and Human Services, Atlanta, GA 30333.

Centers for Disease Control and Prevention .... Jeffrey P. Koplan, M.D., M.P.H.
Director

The material in this report was prepared for publication by
   Epidemiology Program Office .... Stephen B. Thacker, M.D., M.Sc.
Director

      Division of Public Health Surveillance
         and Informatics .... Daniel M. Sosin, M.D., M.P.H.
Director

   National Center for HIV, STD, and TB Prevention .... Helene D. Gayle, M.D., M.P.H.
Director

      Division of HIV/AIDS Prevention —
         Surveillance and Epidemiology .... Robert S. Janssen, M.D.
Director

   National Center for Injury Prevention and Control .... Suzanne Binder, M.D.
Director

   National Center for Chronic Disease Prevention
      and Health Promotion .... James S. Marks, M.D., M.P.H.
Director

      Division of Adult and Community Health .... Gary C. Hogelin, M.P.A.
Director

   National Center for Environmental Health .... Richard J. Jackson, M.D., M.P.H.
Director

      Division of Environmental Hazards and Health Effects .... Michael A. McGeehin
Director

This report was produced as an *MMWR* serial publication in
   Epidemiology Program Office .... Stephen B. Thacker, M.D., M.Sc.
Director

      Office of Scientific and Health Communications .... John W. Ward, M.D.
Director
Editor, MMWR *Series*

          Recommendations and Reports .... Suzanne M. Hewitt, M.P.A.
Managing Editor
Patricia A. McGee
Project Editor
Morie M. Higgins
Visual Information Specialist
Michele D. Renshaw and Erica R. Shaver
Information Technology Specialists

Contents

Guidelines Working Group

CHAIRMAN
Robert R. German, M.P.H.
Epidemiology Program Office, CDC

ADMINISTRATIVE SUPPORT
Dwight Westmoreland, M.P.A.
Epidemiology Program Office, CDC

MEMBERS

Greg Armstrong, M.D.
*National Center for Infectious Diseases
CDC*

Guthrie S. Birkhead, M.D., M.P.H.
Council of State and Territorial
Epidemiologists
*New York State Department of Health
Albany, New York*

John M. Horan, M.D., M.P.H.
*National Center for Injury Prevention
and Control, CDC*

Guillermo Herrera
National Immunization Program, CDC

Lisa M. Lee, Ph.D.
*National Center for HIV, STD and TB
Prevention, CDC*

Robert L. Milstein, M.P.H.
*National Center for Chronic Disease
Prevention and Health Promotion, CDC*

Carol A. Pertowski, M.D.
*National Center for Environmental Health
CDC*

Michael N. Waller
*National Center for Chronic Disease
Prevention and Health Promotion, CDC*

The following CDC staff members prepared this report:

Robert R. German, M.P.H.
Division of Public Health Surveillance and Informatics
Epidemiology Program Office

Lisa M. Lee, Ph.D.
Division of HIV/AIDS Prevention — Surveillance and Epidemiology
National Center for HIV, STD, and TB Prevention

John M. Horan, M.D., M.P.H.
Office of the Director
National Center for Injury Prevention and Control

Robert L. Milstein, M.P.H.
Office of the Director
National Center for Chronic Disease Prevention and Health Promotion

Carol A. Pertowski, M.D.
Division of Environmental Hazards and Health Effects
National Center for Environmental Health

Michael N. Waller
Division of Adult and Community Health
National Center for Chronic Disease Prevention and Health Promotion

in collaboration with

Guthrie S. Birkhead, M.D., M.P.H.
Council of State and Territorial Epidemiologists
New York State Department of Health
Albany, New York

Additional CDC Contributors

Office of the Director: Karen E. Harris, M.P.H.; Joseph A. Reid, Ph.D; Gladys H. Reynolds, Ph.D., M.S.; Dixie E. Snider, Jr., M.D., M.P.H.

Agency for Toxic Substances and Disease Registry: Wendy E. Kaye, Ph.D.; Robert Spengler, Sc.D.

Epidemiology Program Office: Vilma G. Carande-Kulis, Ph.D., M.S.; Andrew G. Dean, M.D., M.P.H.; Samuel L. Groseclose, D.V.M., M.P.H.; Robert A. Hahn, Ph.D., M.P.H.; Lori Hutwagner, M.S.; Denise Koo, M.D., M.P.H.; R. Gibson Parrish, M.D., M.P.H.; Catherine Schenck-Yglesias, M.H.S.; Daniel M. Sosin, M.D., M.P.H.; Donna F. Stroup, Ph.D., M.Sc.; Stephen B. Thacker, M.D., M.Sc.; G. David Williamson, Ph.D.

National Center for Birth Defects and Developmental Disabilities: Joseph Mulnaire, M.D., M.S.P.H.

National Center for Chronic Disease Prevention and Health Promotion: Terry F. Pechacek, Ph.D; Nancy Stroup, Ph.D.

National Center for Environmental Health: Thomas H. Sinks, Ph.D.

National Center for Health Statistics: Jennifer H. Madans, Ph.D.

National Center for HIV, STD, and TB Prevention: James W. Buehler, M.D.; Meade Morgan, Ph.D.

National Center for Infectious Diseases: Janet K. Nicholson, Ph.D; Jose G. Rigau-Perez, M.D., M.P.H.

National Center for Injury Prevention and Control: Richard L. Ehrenberg, M.D.

National Immunization Program: H. Gay Allen, M.S.P.H.; Roger H. Bernier, Ph.D; Nancy Koughan, D.O., M.P.H., M.H.A.; Sandra W. Roush, M.T., M.P.H.

National Institute for Occupational Safety and Health: Rosemary Sokas, M.D., M.O.H.

Public Health Practice Program Office: William A. Yasnoff, M.D., Ph.D.

Consultants and Contributors

Scientific Workgroup on Health-Related Quality of Life Surveillance
St. Louis University, St. Louis, Missouri

Paul Etkind, Dr.P.H., Massachusetts Department of Public Health, Jamaica Plain, Massachusetts; Annie Fine, M.D., New York City Department of Health, New York City, New York; Julie A. Fletcher, D.V.M, M.P.H. candidate, Emory University, Atlanta, Georgia; Daniel J. Friedman, Ph.D., Massachusetts Department of Public Health, Boston, Massachusetts; Richard S. Hopkins, M.D., M.S.P.H., Florida Department of Health, Tallahassee, Florida; Steven C. MacDonald, Ph.D., M.P.H., Washington State Department of Health, Olympia, Washington; Elroy D. Mann, D.V.M., M.Sc., Health Canada, Ottawa, Canada; S. Potjaman, M.D., Government of Thailand, Bangkok, Thailand; Marcel E. Salive, M.D., M.P.H., National Institutes of Health, Bethesda, Maryland.

Updated Guidelines
for Evaluating Public Health Surveillance Systems

Recommendations from the Guidelines Working Group

Summary

The purpose of evaluating public health surveillance systems is to ensure that problems of public health importance are being monitored efficiently and effectively. CDC's Guidelines for Evaluating Surveillance Systems *are being updated to address the need for a) the integration of surveillance and health information systems, b) the establishment of data standards, c) the electronic exchange of health data, and d) changes in the objectives of public health surveillance to facilitate the response of public health to emerging health threats (e.g., new diseases). This report provides updated guidelines for evaluating surveillance systems based on CDC's* Framework for Program Evaluation in Public Health, *research and discussion of concerns related to public health surveillance systems, and comments received from the public health community. The guidelines in this report describe many tasks and related activities that can be applied to public health surveillance systems.*

INTRODUCTION

In 1988, CDC published *Guidelines for Evaluating Surveillance Systems* (*1*) to promote the best use of public health resources through the development of efficient and effective public health surveillance systems. CDC's *Guidelines for Evaluating Surveillance Systems* are being updated to address the need for a) the integration of surveillance and health information systems, b) the establishment of data standards, c) the electronic exchange of health data, and d) changes in the objectives of public health surveillance to facilitate the response of public health to emerging health threats (e.g., new diseases). For example, CDC, with the collaboration of state and local health departments, is implementing the National Electronic Disease Surveillance System (NEDSS) to better manage and enhance the large number of current surveillance systems and allow the public health community to respond more quickly to public health threats (e.g., outbreaks of emerging infectious diseases and bioterrorism) (*2*). When NEDSS is completed, it will electronically integrate and link together several types of surveillance systems with the use of standard data formats; a communications infrastructure built on principles of public health informatics; and agreements on data access, sharing, and confidentiality. In addition, the Health Insurance Portability and Accountability Act of 1996 (HIPAA) mandates that the United States adopt national uniform standards for electronic transactions related to health insurance enrollment and eligibility, health-care encounters, and health insurance claims; for identifiers for health-care providers, payers and individuals, as well as code sets and classification systems used in these transactions; and for security of these transactions (*3*). The electronic exchange of health data inherently involves the protection of patient privacy.

Based on CDC's *Framework for Program Evaluation in Public Health* (*4*), research and discussion of concerns related to public health surveillance systems, and comments received from the public health community, this report provides updated guidelines for evaluating public health surveillance systems.

BACKGROUND

Public health surveillance is the ongoing, systematic collection, analysis, interpretation, and dissemination of data regarding a health-related event for use in public health action to reduce morbidity and mortality and to improve health (*5–7*). Data disseminated by a public health surveillance system can be used for immediate public health action, program planning and evaluation, and formulating research hypotheses. For example, data from a public health surveillance system can be used to

- guide immediate action for cases of public health importance;

- measure the burden of a disease (or other health-related event), including changes in related factors, the identification of populations at high risk, and the identification of new or emerging health concerns;

- monitor trends in the burden of a disease (or other health-related event), including the detection of epidemics (outbreaks) and pandemics;

- guide the planning, implementation, and evaluation of programs to prevent and control disease, injury, or adverse exposure;

- evaluate public policy;

- detect changes in health practices and the effects of these changes;

- prioritize the allocation of health resources;

- describe the clinical course of disease; and

- provide a basis for epidemiologic research.

Public health surveillance activities are generally authorized by legislators and carried out by public health officials. Public health surveillance systems have been developed to address a range of public health needs. In addition, public health information systems have been defined to include a variety of data sources essential to public health action and are often used for surveillance (*8*). These systems vary from a simple system collecting data from a single source, to electronic systems that receive data from many sources in multiple formats, to complex surveys. The number and variety of systems will likely increase with advances in electronic data interchange and integration of data, which will also heighten the importance of patient privacy, data confidentiality, and system security. Appropriate institutions/agencies/scientific officials should be consulted with any projects regarding pubic health surveillance.

Variety might also increase with the range of health-related events under surveillance. In these guidelines, the term "health-related event" refers to any subject related to a public health surveillance system. For example, a health-related event could include infectious, chronic, or zoonotic diseases; injuries; exposures to toxic substances; health promoting or damaging behaviors; and other surveilled events associated with public health action.

The purpose of evaluating public health surveillance systems is to ensure that problems of public health importance are being monitored efficiently and effectively. Public health surveillance systems should be evaluated periodically, and the evaluation should include recommendations for improving quality, efficiency, and usefulness. The goal of these guidelines is to organize the evaluation of a public health surveillance system. Broad topics are outlined into which program-specific qualities can be integrated. Evaluation of a public health surveillance system focuses on how well the system operates to meet its purpose and objectives.

The evaluation of public health surveillance systems should involve an assessment of system attributes, including simplicity, flexibility, data quality, acceptability, sensitivity, predictive value positive, representativeness, timeliness, and stability. With the continuing advancement of technology and the importance of information architecture and related concerns, inherent in these attributes are certain public health informatics concerns for public health surveillance systems. These concerns include comparable hardware and software, standard user interface, standard data format and coding, appropriate quality checks, and adherence to confidentiality and security standards (9). Because public health surveillance systems vary in methods, scope, purpose, and objectives, attributes that are important to one system might be less important to another. A public health surveillance system should emphasize those attributes that are most important for the objectives of the system. Efforts to improve certain attributes (e.g., the ability of a public health surveillance system to detect a health-related event [sensitivity]) might detract from other attributes (e.g., simplicity or timeliness). An evaluation of the public health surveillance system must therefore consider those attributes that are of the highest priority for a given system and its objectives. Considering the attributes that are of the highest priority, the guidelines in this report describe many tasks and related activities that can be applied in the evaluation of public health surveillance systems, with the understanding that all activities under the tasks might not be appropriate for all systems.

Organization of This Report

This report begins with descriptions of each of the tasks involved in evaluating a public health surveillance system. These tasks are adapted from the steps in program evaluation in the *Framework for Program Evaluation in Public Health* (4) as well as from the elements in the original guidelines for evaluating surveillance systems (1). The report concludes with a summary statement regarding evaluating surveillance systems. A checklist that can be detached or photocopied and used when the evaluation is implemented is also included (Appendix A).

To assess the quality of the evaluation activities, relevant standards are provided for each of the tasks for evaluating a public health surveillance system (Appendix B). These standards are adapted from the standards for effective evaluation (i.e., utility, feasibility, propriety, and accuracy) in the *Framework for Program Evaluation in Public Health* (4). Because all activities under the evaluation tasks might not be appropriate for all systems, only those standards that are appropriate to an evaluation should be used.

Task A. Engage the Stakeholders in the Evaluation

Stakeholders can provide input to ensure that the evaluation of a public health surveillance system addresses appropriate questions and assesses pertinent attributes and that its findings will be acceptable and useful. In that context, we define stakeholders as those persons or organizations who use data for the promotion of healthy lifestyles and the prevention and control of disease, injury, or adverse exposure. Those stakeholders who might be interested in defining questions to be addressed by the surveillance system evaluation and subsequently using the findings from it are public health practitioners; health-care providers; data providers and users; representatives of affected communities; governments at the local, state, and federal levels; and professional and private nonprofit organizations.

Task B. Describe the Surveillance System to be Evaluated

Activities

- Describe the public health importance of the health-related event under surveillance.

- Describe the purpose and operation of the system.

- Describe the resources used to operate the system.

Discussion

To construct a balanced and reliable description of the system, multiple sources of information might be needed. The description of the system can be improved by consulting with a variety of persons involved with the system and by checking reported descriptions of the system against direct observation.

B.1. Describe the Public Health Importance of the Health-Related Event Under Surveillance

Definition. The public health importance of a health-related event and the need to have that event under surveillance can be described in several ways. Health-related events that affect many persons or that require large expenditures of resources are of public health importance. However, health-related events that affect few persons might also be important, especially if the events cluster in time and place (e.g., a limited outbreak of a severe disease). In other instances, public concerns might focus attention on a particular health-related event, creating or heightening the importance of an evaluation. Diseases that are now rare because of successful control measures might be perceived as unimportant, but their level of importance should be assessed as a possible sentinel health-related event or for their potential to reemerge. Finally, the public health importance of a health-related event is influenced by its level of preventability (*10*).

Measures. Parameters for measuring the importance of a health-related event—and therefore the public health surveillance system with which it is monitored—can include (7)

- indices of frequency (e.g., the total number of cases and/or deaths; incidence rates, prevalence, and/or mortality rates); and summary measures of population health status (e.g., quality-adjusted life years [QALYS]);

- indices of severity (e.g., bed-disability days, case-fatality ratio, and hospitalization rates and/or disability rates);

- disparities or inequities associated with the health-related event;

- costs associated with the health-related event;

- preventability (10);

- potential clinical course in the absence of an intervention (e.g., vaccinations) (11,12); and

- public interest.

Efforts have been made to provide summary measures of population health status that can be used to make comparative assessments of the health needs of populations (13). Perhaps the best known of these measures are QALYs, years of healthy life (YHLs), and disability-adjusted life years (DALYs). Based on attributes that represent health status and life expectancy, QALYs, YHLs, and DALYs provide one-dimensional measures of overall health. In addition, attempts have been made to quantify the public health importance of various diseases and other health-related events. In a study that describes such an approach, a score was used that takes into account age-specific morbidity and mortality rates as well as health-care costs (14). Another study used a model that ranks public health concerns according to size, urgency, severity of the problem, economic loss, effect on others, effectiveness, propriety, economics, acceptability, legality of solutions, and availability of resources (15).

Preventability can be defined at several levels, including primary prevention (preventing the occurrence of disease or other health-related event), secondary prevention (early detection and intervention with the aim of reversing, halting, or at least retarding the progress of a condition), and tertiary prevention (minimizing the effects of disease and disability among persons already ill). For infectious diseases, preventability can also be described as reducing the secondary attack rate or the number of cases transmitted to contacts of the primary case. From the perspective of surveillance, preventability reflects the potential for effective public health intervention at any of these levels.

B.2. Describe the Purpose and Operation of the Surveillance System

Methods. Methods for describing the operation of the public health surveillance system include

- List the purpose and objectives of the system.

- Describe the planned uses of the data from the system.

- Describe the health-related event under surveillance, including the case definition for each specific condition.

- Cite any legal authority for the data collection.

- Describe where in the organization(s) the system resides, including the context (e.g., the political, administrative, geographic, or social climate) in which the system evaluation will be done.

- Describe the level of integration with other systems, if appropriate.

- Draw a flow chart of the system.

- Describe the components of the system. For example

  — What is the population under surveillance?

  — What is the period of time of the data collection?

  — What data are collected and how are they collected?

  — What are the reporting sources of data for the system?

  — How are the system's data managed (e.g., the transfer, entry, editing, storage, and back up of data)? Does the system comply with applicable standards for data formats and coding schemes? If not, why?

  — How are the system's data analyzed and disseminated?

  — What policies and procedures are in place to ensure patient privacy, data confidentiality, and system security? What is the policy and procedure for releasing data? Do these procedures comply with applicable federal and state statutes and regulations? If not, why?

  — Does the system comply with an applicable records management program? For example, are the system's records properly archived and/or disposed of?

Discussion. The purpose of the system indicates why the system exists, whereas its objectives relate to how the data are used for public health action. The objectives of a public health surveillance system, for example, might address immediate public health action, program planning and evaluation, and formation of research hypotheses (see Background). The purpose and objectives of the system, including the planned uses of its data, establish a frame of reference for evaluating specific components.

A public health surveillance system is dependent on a clear case definition for the health-related event under surveillance (7). The case definition of a health-related event can include clinical manifestations (i.e., symptoms), laboratory results, epidemiologic information (e.g., person, place, and time), and/or specified behaviors, as well as levels of certainty (e.g., confirmed/definite, probable/presumptive, or possible/suspected). The use of a standard case definition increases the specificity of reporting and improves the comparability of the health-related event reported from different sources of data, including geographic areas. Case definitions might exist for a variety of health-related events under surveillance, including diseases, injuries, adverse exposures, and risk factor or protective behaviors. For example, in the United States, CDC and the Council of State and Territorial Epidemiologists (CSTE) have agreed on standard case definitions for selected infectious diseases (16). In addition, CSTE publishes Position Papers that discuss and define a variety of health-related events (17). When possible, a public health surveillance system should use an established case definition, and if it does not, an explanation should be provided.

The evaluation should assess how well the public health surveillance system is integrated with other surveillance and health information systems (e.g., data exchange and sharing in multiple formats, and transformation of data). Streamlining related systems into an integrated public health surveillance network enables individual systems to meet specific data collection needs while avoiding the duplication of effort and lack of standardization that can arise from independent systems (*18*). An integrated system can address comorbidity concerns (e.g., persons infected with human immunodeficiency virus and *Mycobacterium tuberculosis*); identify previously unrecognized risk factors; and provide the means for monitoring additional outcomes from a health-related event. When CDC's NEDSS is completed, it will electronically integrate and link together several types of surveillance activities and facilitate more accurate and timely reporting of disease information to CDC and state and local health departments (*2*).

CSTE has organized professional discussion among practicing public health epidemiologists at state and federal public health agencies. CSTE has also proposed a national public health surveillance system to serve as a basis for local and state public health agencies to a) prioritize surveillance and health information activities and b) advocate for necessary resources for public health agencies at all levels (*19*). This national public health system would be a conceptual framework and virtual surveillance system that incorporates both existing and new surveillance systems for health-related events and their determinants.

Listing the discrete steps that are taken in processing the health-event reports by the system and then depicting these steps in a flow chart is often useful. An example of a simplified flow chart for a generic public health surveillance system is included in this report (Figure 1). The mandates and business processes of the lead agency that operates the system and the participation of other agencies could be included in this chart. The architecture and data flow of the system can also be depicted in the chart (*20,21*). A chart of architecture and data flow should be sufficiently detailed to explain all of the functions of the system, including average times between steps and data transfers.

The description of the components of the public health surveillance system could include discussions related to public health informatics concerns, including comparable hardware and software, standard user interface, standard data format and coding, appropriate quality checks, and adherence to confidentiality and security standards (*9*). For example, comparable hardware and software, standard user interface, and standard data format and coding facilitate efficient data exchange, and a set of common data elements are important for effectively matching data within the system or to other systems.

To document the information needs of public health, CDC, in collaboration with state and local health departments, is developing the Public Health Conceptual Data Model to a) establish data standards for public health, including data definitions, component structures (e.g., for complex data types), code values, and data use; b) collaborate with national health informatics standard-setting bodies to define standards for the exchange of information among public health agencies and health-care providers; and c) construct computerized information systems that conform to established data and data interchange standards for use in the management of data relevant to public health (*22*). In addition, the description of the system's data management might address who is editing the data, how and at what levels the data are edited, and what checks are in place to ensure data quality.

In response to HIPAA mandates, various standard development organizations and terminology and coding groups are working collaboratively to harmonize their separate systems (23). For example, both the Accredited Standards Committee X12 (24), which has dealt principally with standards for health insurance transactions, and Health Level Seven (HL7) (25), which has dealt with standards for clinical messaging and exchange of clinical information with health-care organizations (e.g., hospitals), have collaborated on a standardized approach for providing supplementary information to support health-care claims (26). In the area of classification and coding of diseases and other medical terms, the National Library of Medicine has traditionally provided the Unified Medical Language System, a metathesaurus for clinical coding systems that allows terms in one coding system to be mapped to another (27). The passage of

FIGURE 1. Simplified flow chart for a generic surveillance system

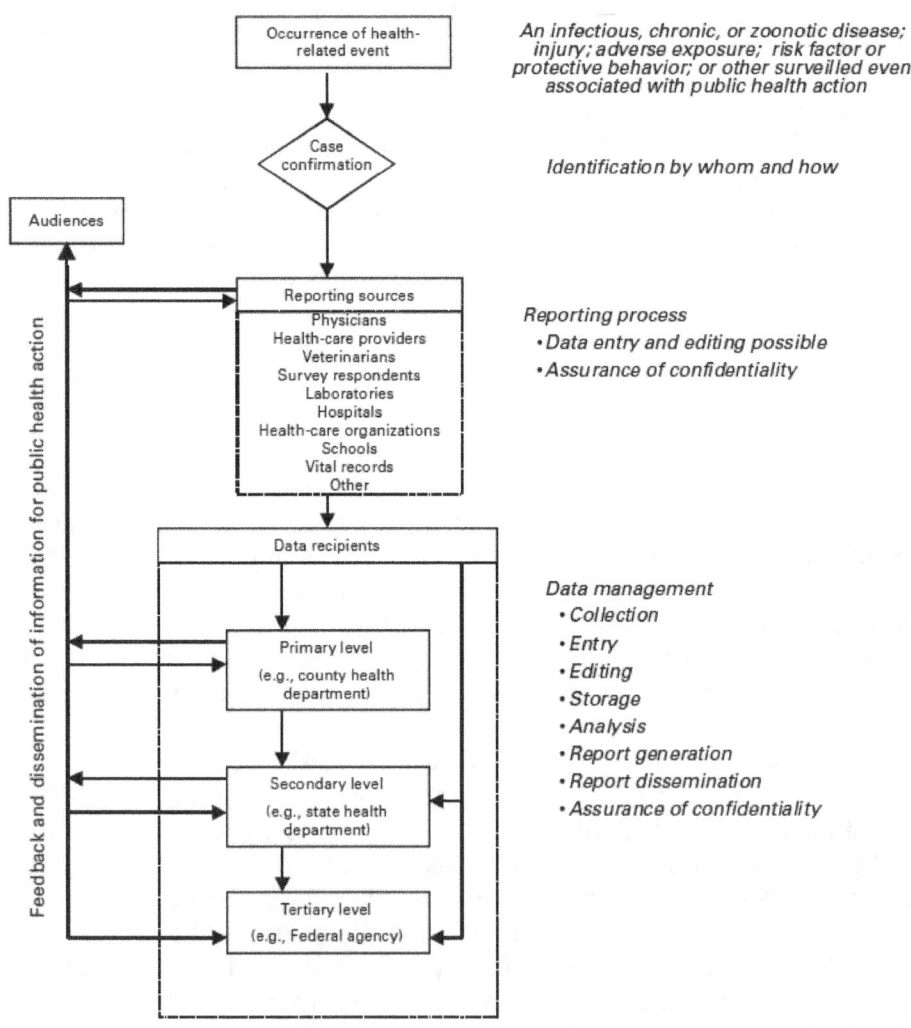

HIPAA and the anticipated adoption of standards for electronic medical records have increased efforts directed toward the integration of clinical terminologies (*23*) (e.g., the merge of the College of American Pathologists' Systematized Nomenclature of Medicine [SNOMED®] [*28*] and the British Read Codes, the National Health Service thesaurus of health-care terms in Great Britain).

The data analysis description might indicate who analyzes the data, how they are analyzed, and how often. This description could also address how the system ensures that appropriate scientific methods are used to analyze the data.

The public health surveillance system should operate in a manner that allows effective dissemination of health data so that decision makers at all levels can readily understand the implications of the information (*7*). Options for disseminating data and/or information from the system include electronic data interchange; public-use data files; the Internet; press releases; newsletters; bulletins; annual and other types of reports; publication in scientific, peer-reviewed journals; and poster and oral presentations, including those at individual, community, and professional meetings. The audiences for health data and information can include public health practitioners, health-care providers, members of affected communities, professional and voluntary organizations, policymakers, the press, and the general public.

In conducting surveillance, public health agencies are authorized to collect personal health data about persons and thus have an obligation to protect against inappropriate use or release of that data. The protection of patient privacy (recognition of a person's right not to share information about him or herself), data confidentiality (assurance of authorized data sharing), and system security (assurance of authorized system access) is essential to maintaining the credibility of any surveillance system. This protection must ensure that data in a surveillance system regarding a person's health status are shared only with authorized persons. Physical, administrative, operational, and computer safeguards for securing the system and protecting its data must allow authorized access while denying access by unauthorized users.

A related concern in protecting health data is data release, including procedures for releasing record-level data; aggregate tabular data; and data in computer-based, interactive query systems. Even though personal identifiers are removed before data are released, the removal of these identifiers might not be a sufficient safeguard for sharing health data. For example, the inclusion of demographic information in a line-listed data file for a small number of cases could lead to indirect identification of a person even though personal identifiers were not provided. In the United States, CDC and CSTE have negotiated a policy for the release of data from the National Notifiable Disease Surveillance System (*29*) to facilitate its use for public health while preserving the confidentiality of the data (*30*). The policy is being evaluated for revision by CDC and CSTE.

Standards for the privacy of individually identifiable health data have been proposed in response to HIPAA (*3*). A model state law has been composed to address privacy, confidentiality, and security concerns arising from the acquisition, use, disclosure, and storage of health information by public health agencies at the state and local levels (*31*). In addition, the Federal Committee on Statistical Methodology's series of *Statistical Policy Working Papers* includes reviews of statistical methods used by federal agencies and their contractors that release statistical tables or microdata files that are collected from persons, businesses, or other units under a pledge of confidentiality. These working papers contain basic statistical methods to limit disclosure (e.g., rules for data suppression to protect privacy and to minimize mistaken inferences from small numbers) and provide recommendations for improving disclosure limitation practices (*32*).

A public health surveillance system might be legally required to participate in a records management program. Records can consist of a variety of materials (e.g., completed forms, electronic files, documents, and reports) that are connected with operating the surveillance system. The proper management of these records prevents a "loss of memory" or "cluttered memory" for the agency that operates the system, and enhances the system's ability to meet its objectives.

B.3. Describe the Resources Used to Operate the Surveillance System

Definition. In this report, the methods for assessing resources cover only those resources directly required to operate a public health surveillance system. These resources are sometimes referred to as "direct costs" and include the personnel and financial resources expended in operating the system.

Methods. In describing these resources consider the following:

- **Funding source(s):** Specify the source of funding for the surveillance system. In the United States, public health surveillance often results from a collaboration among federal, state, and local governments.

- **Personnel requirements:** Estimate the time it takes to operate the system, including the collection, editing, analysis, and dissemination of data (e.g., person-time expended per year of operation). These measures can be converted to dollar estimates by multiplying the person-time by appropriate salary and benefit costs.

- **Other resources:** Determine the cost of other resources, including travel, training, supplies, computer and other equipment, and related services (e.g., mail, telephone, computer support, Internet connections, laboratory support, and hardware and software maintenance).

When appropriate, the description of the system's resources should consider all levels of the public health system, from the local health-care provider to municipal, county, state, and federal health agencies. Resource estimation for public health surveillance systems have been implemented in Vermont (Table 1) and Kentucky (Table 2).

Resource Estimation in Vermont. Two methods of collecting public health surveillance data in Vermont were compared (*33*). The passive system was already in place and consisted of unsolicited reports of notifiable diseases to the district offices or state health department. The active system was implemented in a probability sample of physician practices. Each week, a health department employee called these practitioners to solicit reports of selected notifiable diseases.

In comparing the two systems, an attempt was made to estimate their costs. The estimates of direct expenses were computed for the public health surveillance systems (Table 1).

Resource Estimation in Kentucky. Another example of resource estimation was provided by an assessment of the costs of a public health surveillance system involving the active solicitation of case reports of type A hepatitis in Kentucky (Table 2) (*34*). The resources that were invested into the direct operation of the system in 1983 were for

TABLE 1. Comparison of estimated expenses for health department active and passive surveillance systems — Vermont, June 1, 1980–May 31, 1981*

	Surveillance system	
Expenses	Active[†]	Passive[§]
Paper	$114	$80
Mailing	185	48
Telephone	1,947	175
Personnel		
Secretary	3,000	2,000
Public health nurse	14,025	0
Total	**$19,271**	**$2,303**

*Vogt RL, LaRue D, Klaucke DN, Jillson DA. Comparison of an active and passive surveillance system of primary care providers for hepatitis, measles, rubella, and salmonellosis in Vermont. Am J Public Health 1983;73:795–7.
[†] Active surveillance — weekly calls were made from health departments requesting reports.
[§] Passive surveillance — provider-initiated reporting.

personnel and telephone expenses and were estimated at $3,764 and $535, respectively. Nine more cases were found through this system than would have been found through the passive surveillance system, and an estimated seven hepatitis cases were prevented through administering prophylaxis to the contacts of the nine case-patients.

Discussion. This approach to assessing resources includes only those personnel and material resources required for the operation of surveillance and excludes a broader definition of costs that might be considered in a more comprehensive evaluation. For example, the assessment of resources could include the estimation of indirect costs (e.g., follow-up laboratory tests) and costs of secondary data sources (e.g., vital statistics or survey data).

The assessment of the system's operational resources should not be done in isolation of the program or initiative that relies on the public health surveillance system. A more formal economic evaluation of the system (i.e., judging costs relative to benefits) could be included with the resource description. Estimating the effect of the system on decision making, treatment, care, prevention, education, and/or research might be possible (*35,36*). For some surveillance systems, however, a more realistic approach would be to judge costs based on the objectives and usefulness of the system.

Task C. Focus the Evaluation Design

Definition
The direction and process of the evaluation must be focused to ensure that time and resources are used as efficiently as possible.

Methods
Focusing the evaluation design for a public health surveillance system involves

• determining the specific purpose of the evaluation (e.g., a change in practice);

• identifying stakeholders (Task A) who will receive the findings and recommendations of the evaluation (i.e., the intended users);

TABLE 2. Costs of a 22-week active surveillance program for hepatitis A — Kentucky, 1983*

Activity	Estimated costs
Central office	
Surveillance	
Personnel	$3,764
Telephone	535
Local health offices[†]	
Contact tracing	
Personnel	647
Telephone	149
Travel	31
Contact prophylaxis	
Personnel	469
Immune serum globulin	21
Total	**$5,616**

* Hinds MW, Skaggs JW, Bergeisen GH. Benefit-cost analysis of active surveillance of primary care physicians for hepatitis A. Am J Public Health 1985;75:176–7.

[†] Costs of tracing and providing prophylaxis to 38 additional active surveillance-associated contacts of persons with hepatitis A.

- considering what will be done with the information generated from the evaluation (i.e., the intended uses);

- specifying the questions that will be answered by the evaluation; and

- determining standards for assessing the performance of the system.

Discussion

Depending on the specific purpose of the evaluation, its design could be straightforward or complex. An effective evaluation design is contingent upon a) its specific purpose being understood by all of the stakeholders in the evaluation and b) persons who need to know the findings and recommendations of the design being committed to using the information generated from it. In addition, when multiple stakeholders are involved, agreements that clarify roles and responsibilities might need to be established among those who are implementing the evaluation.

Standards for assessing how the public health surveillance system performs establish what the system must accomplish to be considered successful in meeting its objectives. These standards specify, for example, what levels of usefulness and simplicity are relevant for the system, given its objectives. Approaches to setting useful standards for assessing the system's performance include a review of current scientific literature on the health-related event under surveillance and/or consultation with appropriate specialists, including users of the data.

Task D. Gather Credible Evidence Regarding the Performance of the Surveillance System

Activities

- Indicate the level of usefulness by describing the actions taken as a result of analysis and interpretation of the data from the public health surveillance system. Characterize the entities that have used the data to make decisions and take actions. List other anticipated uses of the data.

- Describe each of the following system attributes:

— Simplicity

— Flexibility

— Data quality

— Acceptability

— Sensitivity

— Predictive value positive

— Representativeness

— Timeliness

— Stability

Discussion

Public health informatics concerns for public health surveillance systems (see Task B.2, Discussion) can be addressed in the evidence gathered regarding the performance of the system. Evidence of the system's performance must be viewed as credible. For example, the gathered evidence must be reliable, valid, and informative for its intended use. Many potential sources of evidence regarding the system's performance exist, including consultations with physicians, epidemiologists, statisticians, behavioral scientists, public health practitioners, laboratory directors, program managers, data providers, and data users.

D.1. Indicate the Level of Usefulness

Definition. A public health surveillance system is useful if it contributes to the prevention and control of adverse health-related events, including an improved understanding of the public health implications of such events. A public health surveillance system can also be useful if it helps to determine that an adverse health-related event previously thought to be unimportant is actually important. In addition, data from a surveillance system can be useful in contributing to performance measures (37), including health indicators (38) that are used in needs assessments and accountability systems.

Methods. An assessment of the usefulness of a public health surveillance system should begin with a review of the objectives of the system and should consider the system's effect on policy decisions and disease-control programs. Depending on the objectives of a particular surveillance system, the system might be considered useful if it satisfactorily addresses at least one of the following questions. Does the system

- detect diseases, injuries, or adverse or protective exposures of public importance in a timely way to permit accurate diagnosis or identification, prevention or treatment, and handling of contacts when appropriate?

- provide estimates of the magnitude of morbidity and mortality related to the health-related event under surveillance, including the identification of factors associated with the event?

- detect trends that signal changes in the occurrence of disease, injury, or adverse or protective exposure, including detection of epidemics (or outbreaks)?

- permit assessment of the effect of prevention and control programs?

- lead to improved clinical, behavioral, social, policy, or environmental practices? or

- stimulate research intended to lead to prevention or control?

A survey of persons who use data from the system might be helpful in gathering evidence regarding the usefulness of the system. The survey could be done either formally with standard methodology or informally.

Discussion. Usefulness might be affected by all the attributes of a public health surveillance system (see Task D.2, Describe Each System Attribute). For example, increased sensitivity might afford a greater opportunity for identifying outbreaks and understanding the natural course of an adverse health-related event in the population under surveillance. Improved timeliness allows control and prevention activities to be initiated earlier. Increased predictive value positive enables public health officials to more accurately focus resources for control and prevention measures. A representative surveillance system will better characterize the epidemiologic characteristics of a health-related event in a defined population. Public health surveillance systems that are simple, flexible, acceptable, and stable will likely be more complete and useful for public health action.

D.2. Describe Each System Attribute

D.2.a. Simplicity

Definition. The simplicity of a public health surveillance system refers to both its structure and ease of operation. Surveillance systems should be as simple as possible while still meeting their objectives.

Methods. A chart describing the flow of data and the lines of response in a surveillance system can help assess the simplicity or complexity of a surveillance system. A simplified flow chart for a generic surveillance system is included in this report (Figure 1).

The following measures (see Task B.2) might be considered in evaluating the simplicity of a system:

- amount and type of data necessary to establish that the health-related event has occurred (i.e., the case definition has been met);

- amount and type of other data on cases (e.g., demographic, behavioral, and exposure information for the health-related event);

- number of organizations involved in receiving case reports;

- level of integration with other systems;

- method of collecting the data, including number and types of reporting sources, and time spent on collecting data;

- amount of follow-up that is necessary to update data on the case;

- method of managing the data, including time spent on transferring, entering, editing, storing, and backing up data;

- methods for analyzing and disseminating the data, including time spent on preparing the data for dissemination;

- staff training requirements; and

- time spent on maintaining the system.

Discussion. Thinking of the simplicity of a public health surveillance system from the design perspective might be useful. An example of a system that is simple in design is one with a case definition that is easy to apply (i.e., the case is easily ascertained) and in which the person identifying the case will also be the one analyzing and using the information. A more complex system might involve some of the following:

- special or follow-up laboratory tests to confirm the case;

- investigation of the case, including telephone contact or a home visit by public health personnel to collect detailed information;

- multiple levels of reporting (e.g., with the National Notifiable Diseases Surveillance System, case reports might start with the health-care provider who makes the diagnosis and pass through county and state health departments before going to CDC [29]); and

- integration of related systems whereby special training is required to collect and/ or interpret data.

Simplicity is closely related to acceptance and timeliness. Simplicity also affects the amount of resources required to operate the system.

D.2.b. Flexibility

Definition. A flexible public health surveillance system can adapt to changing information needs or operating conditions with little additional time, personnel, or allocated funds. Flexible systems can accommodate, for example, new health-related events, changes in case definitions or technology, and variations in funding or reporting sources. In addition, systems that use standard data formats (e.g., in electronic data interchange) can be easily integrated with other systems and thus might be considered flexible.

Methods. Flexibility is probably best evaluated retrospectively by observing how a system has responded to a new demand. An important characteristic of CDC's Behavioral Risk Factor Surveillance System (BRFSS) is its flexibility (*39*). Conducted in collaboration with state health departments, BRFSS is an ongoing sample survey that gathers and reports state-level prevalence data on health behaviors related to the leading preventable causes of death as well as data on preventive health practices. The system permits states to add questions of their own design to the BRFSS questionnaire but is uniform enough to allow state-to-state comparisons for certain questions. These state-specific questions can address emergent and locally important health concerns. In addition, states can stratify their BRFSS samples to estimate prevalence data for regions or counties within their respective states.

Discussion. Unless efforts have been made to adapt the public health surveillance system to another disease (or other health-related event), a revised case definition, additional data sources, new information technology, or changes in funding, assessing the flexibility of that system might be difficult. In the absence of practical experience, the design and workings of a system can be examined. Simpler systems might be more flexible (i.e., fewer components will need to be modified when adapting the system for a change in information needs or operating conditions).

D.2.c. Data Quality

Definition. Data quality reflects the completeness and validity of the data recorded in the public health surveillance system.

Methods. Examining the percentage of "unknown" or "blank" responses to items on surveillance forms is a straightforward and easy measure of data quality. Data of high quality will have low percentages of such responses. However, a full assessment of the completeness and validity of the system's data might require a special study. Data values recorded in the surveillance system can be compared to "true" values through, for example, a review of sampled data (*40*), a special record linkage (*41*), or patient interview (*42*). In addition, the calculation of sensitivity (Task D.2.e) and predictive value positive (Task D.2.f) for the system's data fields might be useful in assessing data quality.

Quality of data is influenced by the performance of the screening and diagnostic tests (i.e., the case definition) for the health-related event, the clarity of hardcopy or electronic surveillance forms, the quality of training and supervision of persons who complete these surveillance forms, and the care exercised in data management. A review of these facets of a public health surveillance system provides an indirect measure of data quality.

Discussion. Most surveillance systems rely on more than simple case counts. Data commonly collected include the demographic characteristics of affected persons, details about the health-related event, and the presence or absence of potential risk factors. The quality of these data depends on their completeness and validity.

The acceptability (see Task D.2.d) and representativeness (Task D.2.g) of a public health surveillance system are related to data quality. With data of high quality, the system can be accepted by those who participate in it. In addition, the system can accurately represent the health-related event under surveillance.

D.2.d. Acceptability

Definition. Acceptability reflects the willingness of persons and organizations to participate in the surveillance system.

Methods. Acceptability refers to the willingness of persons in the sponsoring agency that operates the system and persons outside the sponsoring agency (e.g., persons who are asked to report data) to use the system. To assess acceptability, the points of interaction between the system and its participants must be considered (Figure 1), including persons with the health-related event and those reporting cases.

Quantitative measures of acceptability can include

- subject or agency participation rate (if it is high, how quickly it was achieved);

- interview completion rates and question refusal rates (if the system involves interviews);

- completeness of report forms;

- physician, laboratory, or hospital/facility reporting rate; and

- timeliness of data reporting.

Some of these measures might be obtained from a review of surveillance report forms, whereas others would require special studies or surveys.

Discussion. Acceptability is a largely subjective attribute that encompasses the willingness of persons on whom the public health surveillance system depends to provide accurate, consistent, complete, and timely data. Some factors influencing the acceptability of a particular system are

- the public health importance of the health-related event;

- acknowledgment by the system of the person's contribution;

- dissemination of aggregate data back to reporting sources and interested parties;

- responsiveness of the system to suggestions or comments;

- burden on time relative to available time;

- ease and cost of data reporting;

- federal and state statutory assurance of privacy and confidentiality;

- the ability of the system to protect privacy and confidentiality;

- federal and state statute requirements for data collection and case reporting; and

- participation from the community in which the system operates.

D.2.e. Sensitivity

Definition. The sensitivity of a surveillance system can be considered on two levels. First, at the level of case reporting, sensitivity refers to the proportion of cases of a disease (or other health-related event) detected by the surveillance system (*43*). Second, sensitivity can refer to the ability to detect outbreaks, including the ability to monitor changes in the number of cases over time.

Methods. The measurement of the sensitivity of a public health surveillance system is affected by the likelihood that

- certain diseases or other health-related events are occurring in the population under surveillance;

- cases of certain health-related events are under medical care, receive laboratory testing, or are otherwise coming to the attention of institutions subject to reporting requirements;

- the health-related events will be diagnosed/identified, reflecting the skill of health-care providers and the sensitivity of screening and diagnostic tests (i.e., the case definition); and

- the case will be reported to the system.

These situations can be extended by analogy to public health surveillance systems that do not fit the traditional disease care-provider model. For example, the sensitivity of a telephone-based surveillance system of morbidity or risk factors is affected by

- the number of persons who have telephones, who are at home when the call is placed, and who agree to participate;

- the ability of persons to understand the questions and correctly identify their status; and

- the willingness of respondents to report their status.

The extent to which these situations are explored depends on the system and on the resources available for assessing sensitivity. The primary emphasis in assessing sensitivity — assuming that most reported cases are correctly classified — is to estimate the proportion of the total number of cases in the population under surveillance being detected by the system, represented by A/(A+C) in this report (Table 3).

Surveillance of vaccine-preventable diseases provides an example of where the detection of outbreaks is a critical concern (*44*). Approaches that have been recommended for improving sensitivity of reporting vaccine-preventable diseases might be

TABLE 3. Calculation of sensitivity* and predictive value positive[†] for a surveillance system

Detected by surveillance	Condition present		
	Yes	No	
Yes	True positive A	False positive B	A+B
No	False negative C	True negative D	C+D
	A+C	B+D	Total

* Sensitivity = A/(A+C)
† Predictive value positive (PVP) = A/(A+B)

applicable to other health-related events (*44*). For example, the sensitivity of a system might be improved by

- conducting active surveillance (i.e., contacting all providers and institutions responsible for reporting cases);

- using external standards (or other surveillance indicators) to monitor the quality of case reporting;

- identifying imported cases;

- tracking the number of cases of suspected disease that are reported, investigated, and ruled out as cases;

- monitoring the diagnostic effort (e.g., tracking submission of laboratory requests for diagnostic testing); and

- monitoring the circulation of the agent (e.g., virus or bacterium) that causes the disease.

The capacity for a public health surveillance system to detect outbreaks (or other changes in incidence and prevalence) might be enhanced substantially if detailed diagnostic tests are included in the system. For example, the use of molecular subtyping in the surveillance of *Escherichia coli* O157:H7 infections in Minnesota enabled the surveillance system to detect outbreaks that would otherwise have gone unrecognized (*45*).

The measurement of the sensitivity of the surveillance system (Table 3) requires a) collection of or access to data usually external to the system to determine the true frequency of the condition in the population under surveillance (*46*) and b) validation of the data collected by the system. Examples of data sources used to assess the sensitivity of health information or public health surveillance systems include medical records (*47,48*) and registries (*49,50*). In addition, sensitivity can be assessed through estimations of the total cases in the population under surveillance by using capture-recapture techniques (*51,52*).

To adequately assess the sensitivity of the public health surveillance system, calculating more than one measurement of the attribute might be necessary. For example, sensitivity could be determined for the system's data fields, for each data source or for combinations of data sources (*48*), for specific conditions under surveillance (*53*), or for each of several years (*54*). The use of a Venn diagram might help depict measurements of sensitivity for combinations of the system's data sources (*55*).

Discussion. A literature review can be helpful in determining sensitivity measurements for a public health surveillance system (*56*). The assessment of the sensitivity of each data source, including combinations of data sources, can determine if the elimination of a current data source or if the addition of a new data source would affect the overall surveillance results (*48*).

A public health surveillance system that does not have high sensitivity can still be useful in monitoring trends as long as the sensitivity remains reasonably constant over time. Questions concerning sensitivity in surveillance systems most commonly arise when changes in the occurrence of a health-related event are noted. Changes in sensitivity can be precipitated by some circumstances (e.g., heightened awareness of a health-related event, introduction of new diagnostic tests, and changes in the method of conducting surveillance). A search for such "artifacts" is often an initial step in outbreak investigations.

D.2.f. Predictive Value Positive

Definition. Predictive value positive (PVP) is the proportion of reported cases that actually have the health-related event under surveillance (*43*).

Methods. The assessment of sensitivity and of PVP provide different perspectives regarding how well the system is operating. Depending on the objectives of the public health surveillance system, assessing PVP whenever sensitivity has been assessed might be necessary (*47–50,53*). In this report, PVP is represented by A/(A+B) (Table 3).

In assessing PVP, primary emphasis is placed on the confirmation of cases reported through the surveillance system. The effect of PVP on the use of public health resources can be considered on two levels. At the level of case detection, PVP affects the amount of resources used for case investigations. For example, in some states, every reported case of type A hepatitis is promptly investigated by a public health nurse, and contacts at risk are referred for prophylactic treatment. A surveillance system with low PVP, and therefore frequent "false-positive" case reports, would lead to misdirected resources.

At the level of outbreak (or epidemic) detection, a high rate of erroneous case reports might trigger an inappropriate outbreak investigation. Therefore, the proportion of epidemics identified by the surveillance system that are true epidemics can be used to assess this attribute.

Calculating the PVP might require that records be kept of investigations prompted by information obtained from the public health surveillance system. At the level of case detection, a record of the number of case investigations completed and the proportion of reported persons who actually had the health-related event under surveillance would allow the calculation of the PVP. At the level of outbreak detection, the review of personnel activity reports, travel records, and telephone logbooks might enable the assessment of PVP. For some surveillance systems, however, a review of data external to the system (e.g., medical records) might be necessary to confirm cases to calculate PVP. Examples of data sources used to assess the PVP of health information or public health surveillance systems include medical records (*48,57*), registries (*49,58*), and death certificates (*59*).

To assess the PVP of the system adequately, calculating more than one measurement of the attribute might be necessary. For example, PVP could be determined for the system's data fields, for each data source or combinations of data sources (*48*), or for specific health-related events (*49*).

Discussion. PVP is important because a low value means that noncases might be investigated, and outbreaks might be identified that are not true but are instead artifacts of the public health surveillance system (e.g., a "pseudo-outbreak"). False-positive reports can lead to unnecessary interventions, and falsely detected outbreaks can lead to costly investigations and undue concern in the population under surveillance. A public health surveillance system with a high PVP will lead to fewer misdirected resources.

The PVP reflects the sensitivity and specificity of the case definition (i.e., the screening and diagnostic tests for the health-related event) and the prevalence of the health-related event in the population under surveillance. The PVP can improve with increasing specificity of the case definition. In addition, good communication between the persons who report cases and the receiving agency can lead to an improved PVP.

D.2.g. Representativeness

Definition. A public health surveillance system that is representative accurately describes the occurrence of a health-related event over time and its distribution in the population by place and person.

Methods. Representativeness is assessed by comparing the characteristics of reported events to all such actual events. Although the latter information is generally not known, some judgment of the representativeness of surveillance data is possible, based on knowledge of

- characteristics of the population, including, age, socioeconomic status, access to health care, and geographic location (*60*);

- clinical course of the disease or other health-related event (e.g., latency period, mode of transmission, and outcome [e.g., death, hospitalization, or disability]);

- prevailing medical practices (e.g., sites performing diagnostic tests and physician-referral patterns) (*33,61*); and

- multiple sources of data (e.g., mortality rates for comparison with incidence data and laboratory reports for comparison with physician reports).

Representativeness can be examined through special studies that seek to identify a sample of all cases. For example, the representativeness of a regional injury surveillance system was examined using a systematic sample of injured persons (*62*). The study examined statistical measures of population variables (e.g., age, sex, residence, nature of injury, and hospital admission) and concluded that the differences in the distribution of injuries in the system's database and their distribution in the sampled data should not affect the ability of the surveillance system to achieve its objectives.

For many health-related events under surveillance, the proper analysis and interpretation of the data require the calculation of rates. The denominators for these rate calculations are often obtained from a completely separate data system maintained by another agency (e.g., the United States Bureau of the Census in collaboration with state governments [*63*]). The choice of an appropriate denominator for the rate calculation should be given careful consideration to ensure an accurate representation of the health-related event over time and by place and person. For example, numerators and denominators must be comparable across categories (e.g., race [*64*], age, residence, and/or time period), and the source for the denominator should be consistent over time when measuring trends in rates. In addition, consideration should be given to the selection of the standard population for the adjustment of rates (*65*).

Discussion. To generalize findings from surveillance data to the population at large, the data from a public health surveillance system should accurately reflect the characteristics of the health-related event under surveillance. These characteristics generally relate to time, place, and person. An important result of evaluating the representativeness of a surveillance system is the identification of population subgroups that might be systematically excluded from the reporting system through inadequate methods of monitoring them. This evaluation process enables appropriate modification of data collection procedures and more accurate projection of incidence of the health-related event in the target population (*66*).

For certain health-related events, the accurate description of the event over time involves targeting appropriate points in a broad spectrum of exposure and the resultant disease or condition. In the surveillance of cardiovascular diseases, for example, it might be useful to distinguish between preexposure conditions (e.g., tobacco use policies and social norms), the exposure (e.g., tobacco use, diet, exercise, stress, and genetics), a pre-symptomatic phase (e.g., cholesterol and homocysteine levels), early-staged disease (e.g., abnormal stress test), late-staged disease (e.g., angina and acute myocardial infarction), and death from the disease. The measurement of risk factor behaviors (e.g., tobacco use) might enable the monitoring of important aspects in the development of a disease or other health-related event.

Because surveillance data are used to identify groups at high risk and to target and evaluate interventions, being aware of the strengths and limitations of the system's data is important. Errors and bias can be introduced into the system at any stage (67). For example, case ascertainment (or selection) bias can result from changes in reporting practices over time or from differences in reporting practices by geographic location or by health-care providers. Differential reporting among population subgroups can result in misleading conclusions about the health-related event under surveillance.

D.2.h. Timeliness

Definition. Timeliness reflects the speed between steps in a public health surveillance system.

Methods. A simplified example of the steps in a public health surveillance system is included in this report (Figure 2). The time interval linking any two of these steps can be examined. The interval usually considered first is the amount of time between the onset of a health-related event and the reporting of that event to the public health agency responsible for instituting control and prevention measures. Factors affecting the time involved during this interval can include the patient's recognition of symptoms, the patient's acquisition of medical care, the attending physician's diagnosis or

FIGURE 2. Simplified example of steps in a surveillance system

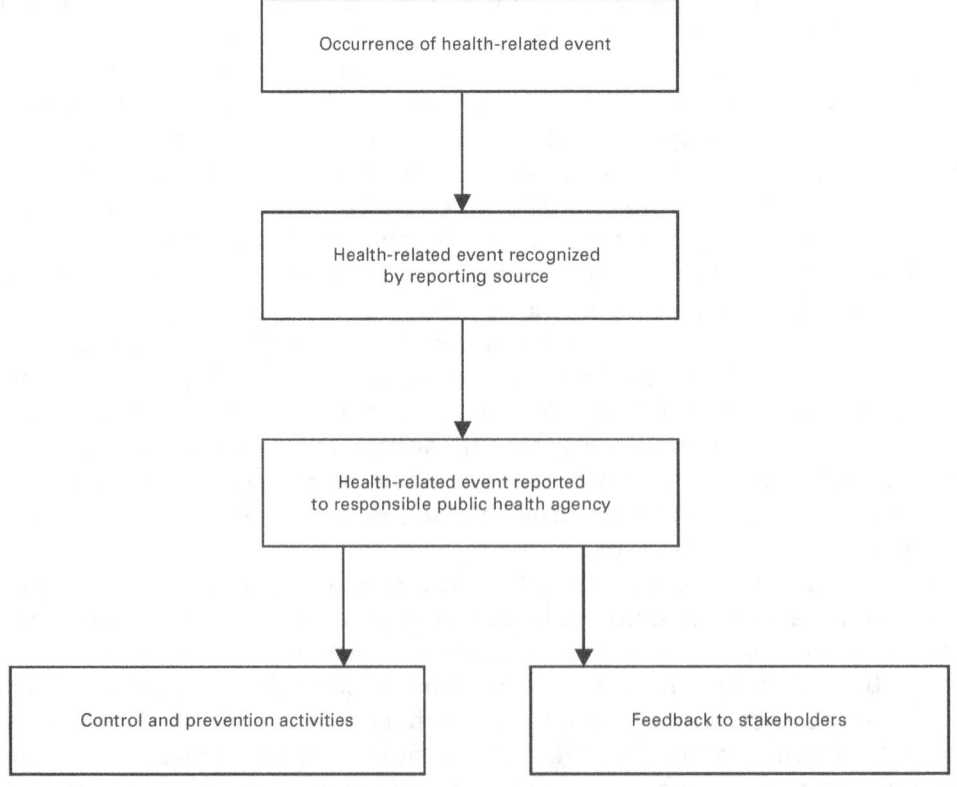

submission of a laboratory test, the laboratory reporting test results back to the physician and/or to a public health agency, and the physician reporting the event to a public health agency. Another aspect of timeliness is the time required for the identification of trends, outbreaks, or the effect of control and prevention measures. Factors that influence the identification process can include the severity and communicability of the health-related event, staffing of the responsible public health agency, and communication among involved health agencies and organizations. The most relevant time interval might vary with the type of health-related event under surveillance. With acute or infectious diseases, for example, the interval from the onset of symptoms or the date of exposure might be used. With chronic diseases, it might be more useful to look at elapsed time from diagnosis rather than from the date of symptom onset.

Discussion. The timeliness of a public health surveillance system should be evaluated in terms of availability of information for control of a health-related event, including immediate control efforts, prevention of continued exposure, or program planning. The need for rapidity of response in a surveillance system depends on the nature of the health-related event under surveillance and the objectives of that system. A study of a public health surveillance system for *Shigella* infections, for example, indicated that the typical case of shigellosis was brought to the attention of health officials 11 days after onset of symptoms — a period sufficient for the occurrence of secondary and tertiary transmission. This example indicates that the level of timeliness was not satisfactory for effective disease control (*68*). However, when a long period of latency occurs between exposure and appearance of disease, the rapid identification of cases of illness might not be as important as the rapid availability of exposure data to provide a basis for interrupting and preventing exposures that lead to disease. For example, children with elevated blood lead levels and no clinically apparent illness are at risk for adverse health-related events. CDC recommends that follow-up of asymptomatic children with elevated blood lead levels include educational activities regarding lead poisoning prevention and investigation and remediation of sources of lead exposure (*69*). In addition, surveillance data are being used by public health agencies to track progress toward national and state health objectives (*38,70*).

The increasing use of electronic data collection from reporting sources (e.g., an electronic laboratory-based surveillance system) and via the Internet (a web-based system), as well as the increasing use of electronic data interchange by surveillance systems, might promote timeliness (*6,29,71,72*).

D.2.i. Stability

Definition. Stability refers to the reliability (i.e., the ability to collect, manage, and provide data properly without failure) and availability (the ability to be operational when it is needed) of the public health surveillance system.

Methods. Measures of the system's stability can include

- the number of unscheduled outages and down times for the system's computer;

- the costs involved with any repair of the system's computer, including parts, service, and amount of time required for the repair;

- the percentage of time the system is operating fully;

- the desired and actual amount of time required for the system to collect or receive data;

- the desired and actual amount of time required for the system to manage the data, including transfer, entry, editing, storage, and back-up of data; and

- the desired and actual amount of time required for the system to release data.

Discussion. A lack of dedicated resources might affect the stability of a public health surveillance system. For example, workforce shortages can threaten reliability and availability. Yet, regardless of the health-related event being monitored, a stable performance is crucial to the viability of the surveillance system. Unreliable and unavailable surveillance systems can delay or prevent necessary public health action.

A more formal assessment of the system's stability could be made through modeling procedures (*73*). However, a more useful approach might involve assessing stability based on the purpose and objectives of the system.

Task E. Justify and State Conclusions, and Make Recommendations

Conclusions from the evaluation can be justified through appropriate analysis, synthesis, interpretation, and judgement of the gathered evidence regarding the performance of the public health surveillance system (Task D). Because the stakeholders (Task A) must agree that the conclusions are justified before they will use findings from the evaluation with confidence, the gathered evidence should be linked to their relevant standards for assessing the system's performance (Task C). In addition, the conclusions should state whether the surveillance system is addressing an important public health problem (Task B.1) and is meeting its objectives (Task B.2).

Recommendations should address the modification and/or continuation of the public health surveillance system. Before recommending modifications to a system, the evaluation should consider the interdependence of the system's costs (Task B.3) and attributes (Task D.2). Strengthening one system attribute could adversely affect another attribute of a higher priority. Efforts to improve sensitivity, PVP, representativeness, timeliness, and stability can increase the cost of a surveillance system, although savings in efficiency with computer technology (e.g., electronic reporting) might offset some of these costs. As sensitivity and PVP approach 100%, a surveillance system is more likely to be representative of the population with the event under surveillance. However, as sensitivity increases, PVP might decrease. Efforts to increase sensitivity and PVP might increase the complexity of a surveillance system — potentially decreasing its acceptability, timeliness, and flexibility. In a study comparing health-department–initiated (active) surveillance and provider-initiated (passive) surveillance, for example, the active surveillance did not improve timeliness, despite increased sensitivity (*61*). In addition, the recommendations can address concerns about ethical obligations in operating the system (*74*).

In some instances, conclusions from the evaluation indicate that the most appropriate recommendation is to discontinue the public health surveillance system; however, this type of recommendation should be considered carefully before it is issued. The cost of renewing a system that has been discontinued could be substantially greater than the cost of maintaining it. The stakeholders in the evaluation should consider relevant public health and other consequences of discontinuing a surveillance system.

Task F. Ensure Use of Evaluation Findings and Share Lessons Learned

Deliberate effort is needed to ensure that the findings from a public health surveillance system evaluation are used and disseminated appropriately. When the evaluation design is focused (Task C), the stakeholders (Task A) can comment on decisions that might affect the likelihood of gathering credible evidence regarding the system's performance. During the implementation of the evaluation (Tasks D and E), considering how potential findings (particularly negative findings) could affect decisions made about the surveillance system might be necessary. When conclusions from the evaluation and recommendations are made (Task E), follow-up might be necessary to remind intended users of their planned uses and to prevent lessons learned from becoming lost or ignored.

Strategies for communicating the findings from the evaluation and recommendations should be tailored to relevant audiences, including persons who provided data used for the evaluation. In the public health community, for example, a formal written report or oral presentation might be important but not necessarily the only means of communicating findings and recommendations from the evaluation to relevant audiences. Several examples of formal written reports of surveillance evaluations have been included in peer-reviewed journals (51,53,57,59,75).

SUMMARY

The guidelines in this report address evaluations of public health surveillance systems. However, these guidelines could also be applied to several systems, including health information systems used for public health action, surveillance systems that are pilot tested, and information systems at individual hospitals or health-care centers. Additional information can also be useful for planning, establishing, as well as efficiently and effectively monitoring a public health surveillance system (6–7).

To promote the best use of public health resources, all public health surveillance systems should be evaluated periodically. No perfect system exists; however, and trade-offs must always be made. Each system is unique and must balance benefit versus personnel, resources, and cost allocated to each of its components if the system is to achieve its intended purpose and objectives.

The appropriate evaluation of public health surveillance systems becomes paramount as these systems adapt to revised case definitions, new health-related events, new information technology (including standards for data collection and sharing), current requirements for protecting patient privacy, data confidentiality, and system security. The goal of this report has been to make the evaluation process inclusive, explicit, and objective. Yet, this report has presented guidelines — not absolutes — for the evaluation of public health surveillance systems. Progress in surveillance theory, technology, and practice continues to occur, and guidelines for evaluating a surveillance system will necessarily evolve.

References
1. CDC. Guidelines for evaluating surveillance systems. MMWR 1988;37(No. S-5).
2. Health Information and Surveillance System Board. Integration Project: National Electronic Disease Surveillance System. Available at <http://www.cdc.gov/od/hissb/act_int.htm>. Accessed May 7, 2001.

3. Department of Health and Human Services. Administrative simplification. Available at <http://aspe.os.dhhs.gov/admnsimp/Index.htm>. Accessed May 7, 2001.
4. CDC. Framework for program evaluation in public health. MMWR 1999;48(RR-11).
5. Thacker SB. Historical development. In: Teutsch SM, Churchill RE, eds. Principles and practice of public health surveillance, 2nd ed. New York, NY: Oxford University Press, 2000.
6. Buehler JW. Surveillance. In: Rothman KJ, Greenland S. Modern epidemiology, 2nd ed. Philadelphia, PA: Lippencott-Raven, 1998.
7. Teutsch SM, Thacker SB. Planning a public health surveillance system. Epidemiological Bulletin: Pan American Health Organization 1995;16:1–6.
8. Thacker SB, Stroup DF. Future directions for comprehensive public health surveillance and health information systems in the United States. Am J Epidemiol 1994;140:383–97.
9. Yasnoff WA, O'Carroll PW, Koo D, Linkins RW, Kilbourne EM. Public health informatics: improving and transforming public health in the information age. J Public Health Management Practice 2000;6:63–71.
10. CDC. An ounce of prevention: what are the returns? 2nd ed. Atlanta, GA: Department of Health and Human Services, CDC, 1999.
11. CDC. Impact of vaccines universally recommended for children—United States, 1990–1998. MMWR 1999;48:243–8.
12. Hinman AR, Koplan JP. Pertussis and pertussis vaccine: reanalysis of benefits, risks, and costs. JAMA 1984;251:3109–13.
13. Institute of Medicine, Committee on Summary Measures of Population Health. In: Field MJ, Gold MR, eds. Summarizing population health: directions for the development and application of population metrics. Washington, DC: National Academy Press, 1998. Available at <http://books.nap.edu/index.html. Accessed February 2001.
14. Dean AG, West DJ, Weir WM. Measuring loss of life, health, and income due to disease and injury. Public Health Rep 1982;97:38–47.
15. Vilnius D, Dandoy S. A priority rating system for public health programs. Public Health Rep 1990;105:463–70.
16. CDC. Case definitions for infectious conditions under public health surveillance. MMWR 1997;46(RR-10).
17. Council of State and Territorial Epidemiologists. Position statements. Available at <http://www.cste.org/position_statements.htm >. Accessed May 7, 2001.
18. Morris G, Snider D, Katz M. Integrating public health information and surveillance systems. J Public Health Management Practice 1996;2:24–7.
19. Meriwether RA. Blueprint for a National Public Health Surveillance System for the 21st century. J Public Health Management Practice 1996;2(4):16–23.
20. Zachman JA. A framework for information systems architecture. IBM Systems J 1987;26(3).
21. Sowa JF, Zachman JA. Extending and formalizing the framework for information systems architecture. IBM Systems J 1992;31(3).
22. Health Information and Surveillance System Board. Public Health Conceptual Data Model (PHCDM). Available at <http://www.cdc.gov/od/hissb/docs/phcdm.htm >. Accessed May 7, 2001.
23. Koo D, Parrish RG II. The changing health-care information infrastructure in the United States: opportunities for a new approach to public health surveillance. In: Teutsch SM, Churchill RE, eds. Principles and practice of public health surveillance, 2nd ed. New York, NY: Oxford University Press, 2000.
24. Data Interchange Standards Association. X12 Standards, release 4020. Alexandria, VA: Accredited Standards Committee X12, 1998. Available at <http://www.disa.org>. Accessed May 7, 2001.
25. Health Level Seven. Available at <http://www.hl7.org >. Accessed May 7, 2001.
26. Health Care Financing Administration. The Health Insurance Portability and Accountability Act of 1996 (HIPAA). Available at <http://www.hcfa.gov/hipaa/hipaahm.htm>. Accessed May 7, 2001.

27. Humphreys BL, Lindberg DAB, Schoolman HM, Barnett GO. The unified medical language system: an informatics research collaboration. JAMIA 1998;5:1–11.

28. College of American Pathologists. Systematized nomenclature of human and veterinary medicine (SNOMED®), version 3.5. Northfield, IL: College of American Pathologists. Available at <http://www.snomed.org/snomed35_txt.html>. Accessed May 7, 2001.

29. Koo D, Wetterhall SF. History and current status of the National Notifiable Diseases Surveillance System. J Public Health Management Practice 1996;2:4–10.

30. Council of State and Territorial Epidemiologists. Data release guidelines of the Council of State and Territorial Epidemiologists for the National Public Health Surveillance System. Atlanta, GA: Council of State and Territorial Epidemiologists, June 1996. Available at <http://www.cste.org/>. Accessed February 2001.

31. Privacy Law Advisory Committee, Model State Public Health Privacy Project. Model state public health privacy act. Washington, DC: Georgetown University Law Center, 1999. Available at <http://www.critpath.org/msphpa/privacy.htm>. Accessed May 7, 2001.

32. Federal Committee on Statistical Methodology, Subcommittee on Disclosure Limitation Methodology. Statistical Policy Working Paper 22: report on statistical disclosure limitation methodology. Washington, DC: Office of Management and Budget, May 1994 (PB94-165305). Available at <http://www.ntis.gov/>. Accessed May 7, 2001.

33. Vogt RL, LaRue D, Klaucke DN, Jillson DA. Comparison of an active and passive surveillance system of primary care providers for hepatitis, measles, rubella, and salmonellosis in Vermont. Am J Public Health 1983;73:795–7.

34. Hinds MW, Skaggs JW, Bergeisen GH. Benefit-cost analysis of active surveillance of primary care physicians for hepatitis A. Am J Public Health 1985;75:176–7.

35. Morris S, Gray A, Noone A, Wiseman M, Jathanna S. The costs and effectiveness of surveillance of communicable disease: a case study of HIV and AIDS in England and Wales. J Public Health Med 1996;18:415–22.

36. Haddix AC, Teutsch SM, Shaffer PA, Duñet, DO, eds. Prevention effectiveness: a guide to decision analysis and economic evaluation. New York, NY: Oxford University Press, 1996.

37. Department of Health and Human Services, Health Resources and Services Administration. Title V (Title V IS) information system web site. Accessed at <http://www.mchdata.net/>. Accessed May 7, 2001.

38. US Department of Health and Human Services. Healthy people 2010 (conference ed, 2 vols). Washington, DC: US Department of Health and Human Services, 2000.

39. Behavioral Risk Factor Surveillance System. Available at <http://www.cdc.gov/nccdphp/brfss/>. Accessed May 7, 2001.

40. Klevens RM, Fleming PL, Neal JJ, Mode of Transmission Validation Study Group. Is there really a heterosexual AIDS epidemic in the United States? Findings from a multisite validation study, 1992-1995. Am J Epidemiol 1999;149:75–84.

41. Fox J, Stahlsmith L, Remington P, Tymus T, Hargarten S. The Wisconsin firearm-related injury surveillance system. Am J Prev Med 1998;15:101–8.

42. Phillips-Howard PA, Mitchell J, Bradley DJ. Validation of malaria surveillance case reports: implications for studies of malaria risk. J Epidemiol Community Health 1990;44:155–61.

43. Weinstein MC, Fineberg HV. Clinical decision analysis. Philadelphia, PA: W.B. Saunders, 1980:84–94.

44. CDC. Manual for the surveillance of vaccine-preventable diseases. Atlanta, GA: Department of Health and Human Services, CDC, September 1999.

45. Bender JB, Hedberg CW, Besser JM, MacDonald KL, Osterholm MT. Surveillance for *Escherichia coli* 0157:H7 infections in Minnesota by molecular subtyping. N Engl J Med 1997;337:388–94.

46. Chandra Sekar C, Deming WE. On a method of estimating birth and death rates and the extent of registration. J Am Stat Assoc 1949;44:101–15.

47. Emori TG, Edwards JR, Culver DH, et al. Accuracy of reporting nosocomial infections in intensive-care–unit patients to the National Nosocomial Infections Surveillance System: a pilot study. Infect Control Hosp Epidemiol 1998;19:308–16.
48. Johnson RL, Gabella BA, Gerhart KA, McCray J, Menconi JC, Whiteneck GG. Evaluating sources of traumatic spinal cord injury surveillance data in Colorado. Am J Epidemiol 1997;146:266–72.
49. Watkins ML, Edmonds L, McClearn A, Mullins L, Mulinare J, Khoury M. The surveillance of birth defects: the usefulness of the revised US standard birth certificate. Am J Public Health 1996;86:731–4.
50. Payne SMC, Seage GR III, Oddleifson S, et al. Using administratively collected hospital discharge data for AIDS surveillance. Ann Epidemiol 1995;5:337–46.
51. Van Tuinen M, Crosby A. Missouri firearm-related injury surveillance system. Am J Prev Med 1998;15:67–74.
52. Hook EB, Regal RR. The value of capture-recapture methods even for apparent exhaustive surveys. Am J Epidemiol 1992;135:1060–7.
53. Gazarian M, Williams K, Elliott E, et al. Evaluation of a national surveillance unit. Arch Dis Child 1999;80:21–7.
54. Singh J, Foster SO. Sensitivity of poliomyelitis surveillance in India. Indian J Pediatr 1998;35:311–5.
55. Last JM, Abramson JH, Friedman GD, Porta M, Spasoff RA, Thuriaux M, eds. A dictionary of epidemiology, 3rd ed. New York, NY: Oxford University Press, 1995:173–4.
56. German RR. Sensitivity and predictive value positive measurements for public health surveillance systems. Epidemiology 2000;11:720–7.
57. Hedegaard H, Wake M, Hoffman R. Firearm-related injury surveillance in Colorado. Am J Prev Med 1998;15(3S):38–45.
58. Mähönen M, Salomaa V, Brommels M, et al. The validity of hospital discharge register data on coronary heart disease in Finland. Eur J Epidemiol 1997;13:403–15.
59. LeMier M, Cummings P, Keck D, Stehr-Green J, Ikeda R, Saltzman L. Washington state gunshot-wound surveillance system. Am J Prev Med 1998;15(3S):92–100.
60. Kimball AM, Thacker SB, Levy ME. Shigella surveillance in a large metropolitan area: assessment of a passive reporting system. Am J Public Health 1980;70:164–6.
61. Thacker SB, Redmond S, Rothenberg RB, Spitz SB, Choi K, White MC. A controlled trial of disease surveillance strategies. Am J Prev Med 1986;2:345–50.
62. McClure RJ, Burnside J. The Australian Capital Territory Injury Surveillance and Prevention Project. Acad Emerg Med 1995;2:529–34.
63. US Bureau of the Census. Federal-State Cooperative Program for Population Estimates: Operational Guidelines. Washington, DC: US Bureau of the Census, July 1992. Available at <http://www.census.gov/population/www/fscpp/fscpp.html>. Accessed February 2001.
64. Hahn RA, Stroup DF. Race and ethnicity in public health surveillance: criteria for the scientific use of social categories. Public Health Rep 1994;109:7–15.
65. CDC. New population standard for age-adjusting death rates. MMWR 1999;48:126–7.
66. Alter MJ, Mares A, Hadler SC, Maynard JE. The effect of underreporting on the apparent incidence and epidemiology of acute viral hepatitis. Am J Epidemiol 1987;125:133–9.
67. Romaguera RA, German RR, Klaucke DN. Evaluating public health surveillance. In: Teutsch SM, Churchill RE, eds. Principles and practice of public health surveillance, 2nd ed. New York, NY: Oxford University Press, 2000.
68. Rosenberg ML. Shigella surveillance in the United States, 1975. J Infect Dis 1977;136:458–60.
69. CDC. Preventing lead poisoning in young children: a statement by the Centers for Disease Control—October 1991. Atlanta, GA: Department of Health and Human Services, Public Health Service, CDC, 1991.

70. Maiese DR. Data challenges and successes with healthy people. Hyattsville, MD: Department of Health and Human Services, CDC, National Center for Health Statistics. Healthy People 2000 Statistics and Surveillance 1998. (no. 9).

71. Effler P, Ching-Lee M, Bogard A, leong M-C, Nekomoto T, Jernigan D. Statewide system of electronic notifiable disease reporting from clinical laboratories: comparing automated reporting with conventional methods. JAMA 1999;282:1845–50.

72. Yokoe DS, Subramanyan GS, Nardell E, Sharnprapai S, McCray E, Platt R. Supplementing tuberculosis surveillance with automated data from health maintenance organizations. Emerg Infect Dis 1999:5:779–87.

73. Johnson AM Jr, Malek M. Survey of software tools for evaluating reliability, availability, and serviceability. Association for Computing Machinery Surveys 1988;20(4).

74. Snider DE, Stroup DF. Ethical issues. In: Teutsch SM, Churchill RE, eds. Principles and practice of public health surveillance, 2nd ed. New York, NY: Oxford University Press, 2000.

75. Singleton JA, Lloyd JC, Mootrey GT, Salive ME, Chen RT, VAERS Working Group. An overview of the vaccine adverse event reporting system (VAERS) as a surveillance system. Vaccine 1999;17:2908–17.

Appendix A.

Checklist for Evaluating Public Health Surveillance Systems

Tasks for evaluating a surveillance system*	Page(s) in this report
Task A. Engage the stakeholders in the evaluation	4
Task B. Describe the surveillance system to be evaluated	4–11
1. Describe the public health importance of the health-related event under surveillance	4– 5
a. Indices of frequency	
b. Indices of severity	
c. Disparities or inequities associated with the health-related event	
d. Costs associated with the health-related event	
e. Preventability	
f. Potential future clinical course in the absence of an intervention	
g. Public interest	
2. Describe the purpose and operation of the surveillance system	5–10
a. Purpose and objectives of the system	
b. Planned uses of the data from the system	
c. Health-related event under surveillance, including case definition	
d. Legal authority for data collection	
e. The system resides where in organization(s)	
f. Level of integration with other systems, if appropriate	
g. Flow chart of system	
h. Components of system	
1) Population under surveillance	
2) Period of time of data collection	
3) Data collection	
4) Reporting sources of data	
5) Data management	
6) Data analysis and dissemination	
7) Patient privacy, data confidentiality, and system security	
8) Records management program	
3. Describe the resources used to operate the surveillance system	10–11
a. Funding source(s)	
b. Personnel requirements	
c. Other resources	
Task C. Focus the evaluation design	11–12
1. Determine the specific purpose of the evaluation	
2. Identify stakeholders who will receive the findings and recommendations of the evaluation	
3. Consider what will be done with the information generated from the evaluation	
4. Specify the questions that will be answered by the evaluation	
5. Determine standards for assessing the performance of the system	
Task D. Gather credible evidence regarding the performance of the surveillance system	13–24
1. Indicate the level of usefulness	13–14
2. Describe each system attribute	14–24
a. Simplicity	
b. Flexibility	
c. Data quality	
d. Acceptability	
e. Sensitivity	
f. Predictive value positive	
g. Representativeness	
h. Timeliness	
i. Stability	
Task E. Justify and state conclusions, and make recommendations	24
Task F. Ensure use of evaluation findings and share lessons learned	25

* Adapted from *Framework for Program Evaluation in Public Health* [CDC. Framework for program evaluation in public health. MMWR 1999;48(RR-11)] and the original guidelines [CDC. Guidelines for evaluating surveillance systems. MMWR 1988;37(No. S-5)].

Appendix B.

Cross-reference of Tasks and Relevant Standards

Tasks for evaluating a surveillance system*	Relevant standards†
Task A. Engage the stakeholders in the evaluation.	**Stakeholder identification.** Persons involved in or affected by the evaluation should be identified so that their needs can be addressed.
	Evaluator credibility. The persons conducting the evaluation should be trustworthy and competent in performing the evaluation to ensure that findings from the evaluation achieve maximum credibility and acceptance.
	Formal agreements. If applicable, all principal parties involved in an evaluation should agree in writing to their obligations (i.e., what is to be done, how, by whom, and when) so that each party must adhere to the conditions of the agreement or renegotiate them.
	Rights of human subjects. The evaluation should be designed and conducted in a manner that respects and protects the rights and welfare of human subjects.
	Human interactions. Evaluators should interact respectfully with other persons associated with an evaluation so that participants are not threatened or harmed.
	Conflict of interest. Conflict of interest should be handled openly and honestly so that the evaluation processes and results are not compromised.
	Metaevaluation. The evaluation should be formatively and summatively evaluated against these and other pertinent standards to guide its conduct appropriately and, on completion, to enable close examination of its strengths and weaknesses by stakeholders.
Task B. Describe the surveillance system to be evaluated.	**Complete and fair assessment.** The evaluation should be complete and fair in its examination and recording of strengths and weaknesses of the system so that strengths can be enhanced and problem areas addressed.
	System documentation. The system being evaluated should be documented clearly and accurately.
	Context analysis. The context in which the system exists should be examined in enough detail to identify probable influences on the system.
	Metaevaluation. The evaluation should be formatively and summatively evaluated against these and other pertinent standards to guide its conduct appropriately and, on completion, to enable close examination of its strengths and weaknesses by stakeholders.
Task C. Focus the evaluation design.	**Evaluation impact.** Evaluations should be planned, conducted, and reported in ways that encourage follow-through by stakeholders to increase the likelihood of the evaluation being used.

Appendix B. — Continued

Cross-reference of Tasks and Relevant Standards

Tasks for evaluating a surveillance system*	Relevant standards[†]
Task C. (*Continued*) Focus the evaluation design.	***Practical procedures.*** Evaluation procedures should be practical while needed information is being obtained to keep disruptions to a minimum.
	Political viability. During the planning and conducting of the evaluation, consideration should be given to the varied positions of interest groups so that their cooperation can be obtained and possible attempts by any group to curtail evaluation operations or to bias or misapply the results can be averted or counteracted.
	Cost-effectiveness. The evaluation should be efficient and produce valuable information to justify expended resources.
	Service orientation. The evaluation should be designed to assist organizations in addressing and serving effectively the needs of the targeted participants.
	Complete and fair assessment. The evaluation should be complete and fair in its examination and recording of strengths and weaknesses of the system so that strengths can be enhanced and problem areas addressed.
	Fiscal responsibility. The evaluator's allocation and expenditure of resources should reflect sound accountability procedures by being prudent and ethically responsible so that expenditures are accountable and appropriate.
	Described purpose and procedures. The purpose and procedures of the evaluation should be monitored and described in enough detail to identify and assess them. The purpose of evaluating a surveillance system is to promote the best use of public health resources by ensuring that only important problems are under surveillance and that surveillance systems operate efficiently.
	Metaevaluation. The evaluation should be formatively and summatively evaluated against these and other pertinent standards to guide its conduct appropriately and, on completion, to enable close examination of its strengths and weaknesses by stakeholders.
Task D. Gather credible evidence regarding the performance of the surveillance system.	***Information scope and selection.*** Information collected should address pertinent questions regarding the system and be responsive to the needs and interests of clients and other specified stakeholders.
	Defensible information sources. Sources of information used in the system evaluation should be described in enough detail to assess the adequacy of the information.

Appendix B. — Continued

Cross-reference of Tasks and Relevant Standards

Tasks for evaluating a surveillance system*	Relevant standards[†]
Task D. (*Continued*) Gather credible evidence regarding the performance of the surveillance system.	*Valid information.* Information-gathering procedures should be developed and implemented to ensure a valid interpretation for the intended use. *Reliable information.* Information-gathering procedures should be developed and implemented to ensure sufficiently reliable information for the intended use. *Systematic information.* Information collected, processed, and reported in an evaluation should be systematically reviewed and any errors corrected. *Metaevaluation.* The evaluation should be formatively and summatively evaluated against these and other pertinent standards to guide its conduct appropriately and, on completion, to enable close examination of its strengths and weaknesses by stakeholders.
Task E. Justify and state conclusions, and make recommendations.	*Values identification.* The perspectives, procedures, and rationale used to interpret the findings should be carefully described so that the bases for value judgments are clear. *Analysis of information.* Information should be analyzed appropriately and systematically so that evaluation questions are answered effectively. *Justified conclusions.* Conclusions that are reached should be explicitly justified for stakeholders' assessment. *Metaevaluation.* The evaluation should be formatively and summatively evaluated against these and other pertinent standards to guide its conduct appropriately and, on completion, to enable close examination of its strengths and weaknesses by stakeholders.
Task F. Ensure use of evaluation findings and share lessons learned.	*Evaluator credibility.* The persons conducting the evaluation should be trustworthy and competent in performing the evaluation to ensure that findings from the evaluation achieve maximum credibility and acceptance. *Report clarity.* Evaluation reports should clearly describe the system being evaluated, including its context and the purposes, procedures, and findings of the evaluation so that essential information is provided and easily understood. *Report timeliness and dissemination.* Substantial interim findings and evaluation reports should be disseminated to intended users so that they can be used in a timely fashion.

Appendix B. — Continued

Cross-reference of Tasks and Relevant Standards

Tasks for evaluating a surveillance system*	Relevant standards[†]
Task F. Ensure use of the findings of the evaluation and share lessons learned.	*Evaluation impact.* Evaluations should be planned, conducted, and reported in ways that encourage follow-through by stakeholders to increase the likelihood of the evaluation being used. *Disclosure of findings.* The principal parties of an evaluation should ensure that the full evaluation findings with pertinent limitations are made accessible to the persons affected by the evaluation and any others with expressed legal rights to receive the results. *Impartial reporting.* Reporting procedures should guard against the distortion caused by personal feelings and biases of any party involved in the evaluation so that the evaluation reflects the findings fairly. *Metaevaluation.* The evaluation should be formatively and summatively evaluated against these and other pertinent standards to guide its conduct appropriately and, on completion, to enable close examination of its strengths and weaknesses by stakeholders.

* Adapted from *Framework for Program Evaluation in Public Health* [CDC. Framework for program evaluation in public health. MMWR 1999;48(RR–11)] and the original guidelines [CDC. Guidelines for evaluating surveillance systems. MMWR 1988;37(No. S-5)].

[†] Adapted from *Framework for Program Evaluation in Public Health* [CDC. Framework for program evaluation in public health. MMWR 1999;48(RR-11)].

REFERENCES

1. CDC. Public health surveillance. In: Principles of epidemiology: an introduction to applied epidemiology and biostatistics. Atlanta (GA): Centers for Disease Control and Prevention; 1992. p. 289–345.

2. Wetterhall SF, Pappaioanou M, Thacker SB, Baker E, Churchill RE. The role of public health surveillance: information for effective action in public health. MMWR 1992;41:S207–S218.

3. Bettcher DW, Sapirie S, Goon EH. Essential public health functions: results of the international Delphi study. World Health Stat Q 1994;51:44–54.

4. Buehler JW. Surveillance. In: Rothman KJ, Greenland S, editors. Modern epidemiology. Philadelphia: Lippincott-Raven Publishers; 1998. p. 435–57.

5. Snider DE, Stroup DF. Ethical issues. In: Teutsch SM, Churchill RE, editors. Principles and practice of public health surveillance. New York: Oxford University Press; 2000. p. 194–214.

6. Fathalla M. Reproductive health: a global overview. Ann NY Acad Sci 1991;626:1.

7. Berg C, Danel I, Mora G, editors. Guidelines for maternal mortality epidemiological surveillance. Washington: The World Bank; 1996.

8. Greenberg RS, editor. Medical epidemiology. Norwalk (CT): Appleton and Lange; 1993.

9. Colley Gilbert B, Shulman HB, Fischer LA, Rogers MM. The Pregnancy Risk Assessment Monitoring System (PRAMS): methods and 1996 response rates from 11 states. Matern Child Health J 1999;3:199–209.

10. CDC. Sentinel Surveillance System for antimicrobial resistance in clinical isolates of Neisseria gonorrhoeae. MMWR 1997;36: 585–6, 591–3.

11. Stroup NE, Zack MM, Wharton M. Sources of routinely collected data for surveillance. In: Teutsch SM, Churchill RE, editors. Principles and practice of public health surveillance. New York: Oxford University Press; 1994. p. 31–82.

12. Murray CJ, Lopez AD. Mortality by cause for eight regions of the world: global burden of disease study. Lancet 1997;349: 1269–76.

13. Thacker SB, Berkelman RL. Public health surveillance in the United States. Epidemiol Rev 1988;10:164–90.

14. Stanton C, Abderrahim N, Hill K. DHS maternal mortality indicators: an assessment of data quality and implications for data use. DHS Analytical Reports No. 4. Calverton (MD): Macro International Inc.

15. Safe motherhood indicators—lessons learned in measuring progress. MotherCare Matters 1999;8(1):1–24.

16. Reproductive health in refugee situations: an inter-agency field manual. Geneva, Switzerland: United Nations High Commissioner for Refugees; 1999.

17. White ME, McDonnell SM. Public health surveillance in low- and middle-income countries. In: Teutsch SM, Churchill RE, editors. Principles and practice of public health surveillance. 2nd ed. New York: Oxford University Press; 2000.

18. Teutsch SM. Considerations in planning a surveillance system. In: Teutsch SM, Churchill RE, editors. Principles and practice of public health surveillance. 2nd ed. New York: Oxford University Press; 2000. p. 17–29.

19. Friede A, Blum HL, McDonald M. Public health informatics: how information-age technology can strengthen public health. Annu Rev Public Health 1995;16:239–52.

20. Kilbourne EM. Informatics in public health surveillance: current issues and future perspectives. MMWR 1992;41:S91–S99.

21. Groseclose SL, Sullivan KM, Gibbs NP, Knowles CM. Management of the surveillance information system and quality control of data. In: Teutsch SM, Churchill RE, editors. Principles and practice of public health surveillance. 2nd ed. New York: Oxford University Press; 2000. p. 95–111.

22. Janes GR, Hutwagner LC, Cates W Jr, Stroup DF, Williamson GD. Descriptive epidemiology: analyzing and interpreting surveillance data. In: Teutsch SM, Churchill RE, editors. Principles and practice of public health surveillance. 2nd ed. New York: Oxford University Press; 2000. p. 112–67.

23. CDC. Updated guidelines for evaluating public health surveillance systems: recommendations from the guidelines working group. MMWR 2001;50(No. RR-13):1–35.

24. Padian NS, Washington AE. Pelvic inflammatory disease: a brief overview. Ann Epidemiol 1994;4(2):128–32.

25. Wasserheit JN. Pelvic inflammatory disease and infertility. Md Med J 1987;36(1):58–63.

26. Medecins Sans Frontieres. Refugee health: an approach to emergency situations. London: Macmillan; 1997.

27. Hakewill PA, Moren A. Monitoring and evaluation of relief programmes. Trop Doct 1991;21(Suppl 1):24–8.

28. CDC. Sexually transmitted diseases treatment guidelines, 2002. MMWR 2002;51(No. RR-06):1-80.

www.ingramcontent.com/pod-product-compliance
Lightning Source LLC
Chambersburg PA
CBHW080256180526
45167CB00006B/2549